Infant Crying, Feeding and Sleeping

THE DEVELOPING BODY AND MIND

Series Editor:
Professor George Butterworth, *Department of Psychology, University of Sussex*

Designed for a broad readership in the English-speaking world, this major series represents the best of contemporary research and theory in the cognitive, social, abnormal and biological areas of development.

Infant Crying, Feeding and Sleeping

Development, Problems and Treatments

Edited by

Ian St. James-Roberts,
Gillian Harris
and
David Messer

HARVESTER
WHEATSHEAF

New York   London   Toronto   Sydney   Tokyo   Singapore

First published 1993 by
Harvester Wheatsheaf
Campus 400, Maylands Avenue
Hemel Hempstead
Hertfordshire, HP2 7EZ
A division of
Simon & Schuster International Group

Typeset in $10\frac{1}{2}$/12 pt Ehrhardt
by Vision Typesetting, Manchester

Printed and bound in Great Britain by
BPCC Wheatons Ltd, Exeter

British Library Cataloguing in Publication Data

A catalogue record for this book is available from
the British Library

ISBN 0-7450-1248-5

1 2 3 4 5   97 96 95 94 93

Contents

Introduction

Ian St. James-Roberts, Gillian Harris *and* David Messer

Problems with infant crying, sleeping and feeding are a common source of concern for parents. The exact rate of such problems varies depending on how they are defined, but recent surveys suggest that as many as 1 in 4 families experience such problems, and 1 in 5 seek help from their community health services because of them (Butler and Golding, 1986; Forsyth *et al.*, 1985; Pollock, 1992; St. James-Roberts and Halil, 1991). As a result, the problems are also 'costly' ones for the health services, in the sense that they take up a great deal of professional time. In some cases, the problems are probably transitory and will subside with the minimum of intervention. In other cases, however, they may be part of a more pervasive and protracted disturbance. If the health services are to work effectively, they need ways of distinguishing between these two possibilities. In turn, this requires standard and robust methods of assessment, together with knowledge about longer-term outcomes and the effectiveness of interventions in remedying these.

This book is the result of an expert study group set up by the Association for Child Psychology and Psychiatry to examine these issues. At first sight, it may seem surprising that a group made up predominantly of psychologists and psychiatrists should be involved with problems which have traditionally been seen as a part of primary medical care. There are two main reasons why this has come about.

The first is that crying, feeding and sleeping problems are principally disturbances of *behaviour*, rather than medical conditions. It follows that, as well as physiological disorders, learning and social-interactional processes need to be taken into account in explaining them. The view of infancy proposed in this book is one principally of rapid change and adjustment.

1

During their first year, infants have to achieve a major feat of adaptation, going from an initial 4-hour sleep–waking and feeding cycle to a diurnally organised 24-hour one, and from frequent liquid feeds to infrequent solid meals. At the same time, the infant's psychological repertoire increases enormously in complexity, with the rapid development of learning, cognitive, emotional and motoric abilities and the acquisition of rudimentary social understanding. The infant's task, then, is primarily one of organisation and regulation, that is, of adjusting to and integrating the rapid changes taking place both in internal, physiological and mental systems and in external demands.

Given the extraordinary pace and complexity of development during this period, it is hardly surprising that minor setbacks should be common – indeed, they can be viewed as a normal part of development. Equally, it follows that research and practice need to focus on the qualities which enable adjustment to be made in many cases and which prevent this from happening in others. In turn, this implies the need for a developmental approach, which follows infant problems and adjustments over time, rather than treating them as static disturbances. This developmental approach is a major feature of this book.

The second characteristic of this book's approach is to view crying, feeding and sleeping problems as social, as well as infant, phenomena. In one sense, this is uncontroversial, since infancy involves a special, almost symbiotic, relationship between child and parents. Perhaps more than in any other period of life, infant development depends on outside regulation, so that parents have to provide the resources and support the infant needs and, at the same time, to foster the gradual development of autonomous self-control. Nor is it infants alone who have to make major adjustments during this period; just about every aspect of parental and household life will need to be modified and re-ordered in the months after the birth to take account of the new family structure. It follows that a close understanding of the role of infant–parent interactions in guiding development is a prerequisite of scientific progress – and effective practice – in this area.

As well as providing support for infant development, parents are also a part of infant behaviour problems in a second sense, since it is parents who become concerned about infant behaviour and who seek professional assistance as a result. In effect, behaviour problems have two elements. First, there is an implication that the infant's behaviour is abnormal, due to a disturbance of some kind. Confirmation that this is the case requires objective measures of the behaviour in question, together with comparable figures for the normal range of the behaviour among infants generally. Second, the term behaviour 'problem' goes beyond a mere quantification of behaviour to include a social judgement that the behaviour is unacceptable in a particular context or way. Since such judgements are subjective in nature, they have often been treated with a degree of scepticism – leading to the inference that infant crying, feeding and sleeping are problems for parents rather than for infants. Yet, it is equally true that parents are often sensitive and astute observers of their infants' disturbances.

The approach to this issue adopted here is to accept that infant crying, feeding and sleeping problems are partly social in nature. It follows that one aim for research and practice is to understand the bases for parents' concerns. For example, it is reasonable to expect cultural variations in what is regarded as normal, as well as variations between families within a given culture. At the same time, it is equally important to be able to measure infant behaviour accurately, in order to know whether the behaviour does exhibit disturbances, and to distinguish between the behaviour and parents' impressions of and concerns about it. Indeed, for therapeutic purposes, it will often be the juxtaposition of these different types of information which will be of the greatest value.

These two aims – of understanding infant crying, feeding and sleeping as developmental and as social, as well as medical, phenomena – are central concerns for this book. A third aim is to bring the three areas together and to examine the relationships between them. Perhaps because infant behaviour is of interest to a variety of different professions, the research evidence on crying, feeding and sleeping is scattered across a wide array of journals and books. Yet, it was the shared impression among members of the study group – and much of the impetus for their coming together – that problems in the three areas were often seen together within the same infant.

This fragmentation of infant behaviour problems stands in marked contrast to the situation with older children, where it has long been accepted that disturbances in several areas of behaviour often occur together, implying the existence of a common underlying cause. An important first step for the infant period is therefore to bring the findings for crying, feeding and sleeping together in one place, so that communalities and distinctions can be explored.

In practice, the goal of integrating the three areas is less simple than it sounds, since each area of knowledge has its own structure and conventions, making it difficult to superimpose a single framework. The approach adopted for this book is therefore to recognise these boundaries, by dividing the book into three main parts. Within each part, each group of authors sets out to review what is known about the normal course of development, the nature and causes of problems, and the effectiveness of alternative treatments, for that area of behaviour. A final chapter then has the aim both of identifying links between the areas and of indicating how these bear upon research and practice.

The fourth and final aim of this book is to provide an up-to-date review of research into infant crying, feeding and sleeping problems which will be useful to professionals who work with young children and their families. To this end, workshops together with the primary healthcare professionals involved – in the United Kingdom mainly health visitors and family doctors, together with smaller numbers of social workers, paediatricians, clinical psychologists and psychotherapists – were held in London and Edinburgh, and the resulting feedback has been incorporated into this book.

This is not to say that the book provides a direct 'how to do it' guide for practice in this area. In its present stage of development, the field is some way from providing a small set of recognised intervention strategies – and indeed, the complexity of the area is such that it is uncertain whether such a digest will be possible in the forseeable future. Rather, what the book sets out to do is to provide an overall grasp of the findings together with some general principles, which will help to guide practitioners in making assessments and in identifying the most effective strategies to adopt in managing individual cases. We believe that a knowledge of developmental and social processes is essential for effective practice in this area. In turn, a better knowledge of the properties of effective treatments will feed back on and enrich our theoretical understanding of the nature of infant development.

References

Butler, N.R. and Golding, J. (1986), *From Birth To Five* (Oxford: Pergamon Press).

Forsyth, B.W.C., Leventhal, J.M. and McCarthy, P.L. (1985), 'Mothers' perceptions of problems of feeding and crying behaviors: a prospective study', *American Journal of Disease in Childhood*, 139, pp. 269–72.

Pollock, J.I. (1992), 'Predictors and long term associations of reported sleeping difficulties in infancy', *Journal of Reproductive and Infant Psychology*, 10, pp. 151–68.

St. James-Roberts, I. and Halil, T. (1991), 'Infant crying patterns in the first year: normative and clinical findings', *Journal of Child Psychology and Psychiatry*, 32, pp. 951–68.

Part 1

Crying

Chapter 1

Infant crying: normal development and persistent crying

Ian St. James-Roberts, *University of London*

Scope and definition

Infant crying can be studied for a variety of reasons. For instance, cry quality has been examined both as a possible measure of cerebral dysfunction (Zeskind and Lester, 1978) and by researchers interested in the precursors of language development (Lieberman, 1985). In contrast, the main focus of the present review will be on the *amount* that infants cry. One reason for this focus is practical, since persistent infant crying is a common source of parental distress and an element in some cases of infant abuse (Forsyth *et al.*, 1985; Frodi, 1985). Since the crying leads many parents to seek professional assistance, it is also a major and costly element in professional caseloads at a time of increasing concern about the cost-effectiveness of the health services (St. James-Roberts, 1991, 1992a). As well as such practical concerns, there are also theoretical reasons for studying variations in the amounts infants cry. Researchers interested, for instance, in the theoretical concepts of temperament and attachment are drawn to crying because its study can throw light on the contribution of infant and parents to early behaviour disturbances (Bell and Ainsworth, 1972; Hubbard and van IJzendoorn, 1987; St. James-Roberts and Wolke, 1988).

The aim of measuring how much infants cry is a deceptively simple one. In practice, two main pitfalls have come to light. The first is the apparent, but easily overlooked, fact that it is parental complaints of excessive infant crying which are the presenting clinical phenomenon, rather than infant crying itself. For clinical purposes, it is therefore important to understand how parents perceive infant crying and how it affects them, as well as to understand the actual crying. Related to this, the second pitfall is the lack of agreed criteria and methods to define what crying is. Perhaps because crying seems such a straightforward concrete phenomenon, no sustained effort has been made to delineate what is, and is not, denoted by the term. Most dictionary definitions of crying refer to 'distressed vocalisations', so that techniques which capture audible sounds appear on the face of it to be the methods of choice. However, where parents have kept diaries of 'crying', much of the behaviour which concerns them is irritable 'fretting' or 'fussing', only part of which is of an audible kind (Barr et al., 1988; St. James-Roberts, 1992b). One way round this is to distinguish two separate 'crying' states: crying, and 'fretting' or 'fussing', and some researchers have made this distinction using both audible and visible behaviours (Hopkins and van Wulfften-Palthe, 1987; Prechtl, 1974; Wolff, 1987). However, there is little consensus among researchers generally as to whether such a simple dichotomous distinction is a valid one. Some have argued that crying is a continuous graded signal, representing an undifferentiated continuum of distressed arousal, rather than two discrete states (Zeskind et al., 1985). Others, in contrast, have proposed the existence of three crying types: hunger, pain and frustration (Wasz-Hockert et al., 1985), or have distinguished up to twelve different categories of distressed behaviour (Thompson and Lamb, 1983).

These definitional and methodological issues are highlighted at the start of this chapter, since there is already evidence that more or less inclusive definitions produce substantially different figures for the amounts infants cry (Barr et al., 1988; St. James-Roberts et al., 1993). In the longer term, the need is for greater standardisation of criteria and methods and there are signs of some initial attempts towards this goal (Barr and Desilets, 1992; St. James-Roberts et al., 1991). In the meantime, the lack of standardisation makes any attempt to summarise across studies, such as the present one, a hazardous undertaking. Wherever possible, the approach adopted will be to acknowledge the definitional and methodological constraints of the studies as they are discussed. Since infant crying is often taken as a sign of feeding or sleeping problems, this chapter's main goal will be to summarise what is known about crying and its development in normal and referred groups, so that feeding, sleeping and other explanations of the crying can be explored. Bearing in mind the clinical significance of infant crying, the second aim will be to assess what is known about the relationship between infant crying and its impact on parents and the community more generally.

Infant crying in western communities

It seems surprising that, until recently, few figures have been available to show how much infants in the normal community cry. Such normative figures are essential in deciding how much crying is 'excessive'. Ideally, too, primary healthcare staff should have the figures at their fingertips, so that they can reassure parents that certain amounts and patterns of crying are common, or seek specialist referral where this is justified. Accurate figures should also help the professionals to target the individuals most in need of assistance and so enable them to plan the most effective use of their resources.

Figure 1.1 summarises the amounts of daily crying found by studies in the United States, Canada, England and Finland. An important proviso is that most of these figures stem from maternal diaries or questionnaires and relate to overall measures of crying and fussing, rather than attempting to distinguish between these. The agreement between the figures from different studies and countries is, however, sufficient to suggest that they represent reasonably accurate accounts of distressed infant behaviour in western communities. In addition, there is objective confirmation for some of the figures, based on 24-hour audiotape recordings. The following conclusions seem justified:

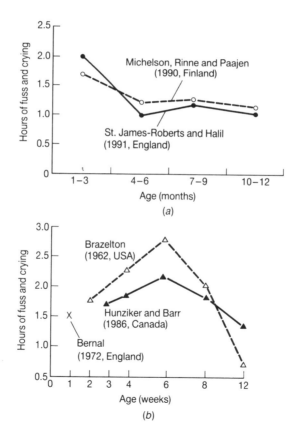

Figure 1.1 Average amount of fuss/crying per 24 hours at different ages. (a) Per quarter year, (b) within the first three months.

1. Infants cry most in the first three months, following which crying declines to about half its earlier level (Fig. 1.1 (*a*)). Broadly speaking, mothers in Canada, England and the United States report that their infants fuss and cry an average of two hours or so per day during the first three months and comparable levels have been found using 24-hour audiotape recordings (St. James-Roberts *et al.*, 1993). Michelsson *et al.* (1990) did not specify the precise method they used in measuring crying, so that their slightly lower 24-hour total (1.6 hours) may be due to method/definitional factors or to lower crying levels in Finland. In England, mothers reported average crying levels of approximately one hour per day (54–72 minutes) for 4–12-month-old infants (St. James-Roberts and Halil, 1991), with similar levels found in Finland (Michelsson *et al.*, 1990).

2. Perhaps unexpectedly, crying is not at a maximum in the newborn period. Rather, most studies show a progressive increase from birth until around the age of six weeks, followed by a decline (Fig. 1.1 (*b*); see, too, Barr (1990)). It is important to note that there is considerable individual variability in the precise age of this 'developmental crying peak', with some infants peaking earlier and some beyond six weeks (Barr, 1990).

3. Changes of daily crying *pattern* also occur with age. As Fig. 1.2 shows, the decline in overall crying beyond three months is due to reductions in amounts of crying in the morning, afternoon and evening. Especially striking, however, is the initial predominance of evening crying, which accounts for some 40 per cent of the daily crying total during the first three months (Barr, 1990; St. James-Roberts and Halil, 1991). St. James-Roberts *et al.* (1993) have found confirmatory evidence of this time-of-day crying 'peak' using tape recordings. Noteworthy is that this evening crying peak in the first three months is common: 49 per cent of Northamptonshire mothers reported an evening peak to their infants' daily crying patterns, with a further 21 per cent reporting a peak in the afternoon (St. James-Roberts and Halil, 1991). Beyond three months, evening crying declines markedly, so that crying over the different periods of the day evens out in the middle of the first year (Fig. 1.2). At approximately nine months of age, St. James-Roberts and Halil (1991) reported a second change of crying pattern, such that night-time crying became more common. Unlike the evening peak in the first three months, night-time crying at 9–12 months occurred predominantly in infants who cried above mean levels generally.

As indicated earlier, the measures of infant crying used in these studies are summaries of overall crying and fussing behaviour. However, two recent studies, both using maternal diaries, have attempted to distinguish whether the crying peaks in the first three months are made up mainly of fussing or crying (Barr, Desilets and Rotman 1991a; St. James-Roberts *et al.*, 1991). Both studies reported that the evening peak, in particular, consists predominantly of fussing. In view of the confusion surrounding the definition of fussing, this finding must be interpreted with some caution. A conservative

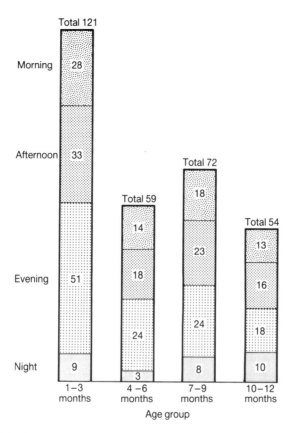

Figure 1.2 Crying patterns at different ages: average amounts of fuss/crying in the morning (6 am–12 am), afternoon (12 am–6 pm), evening (6 pm–12 pm), night (12 pm–6 am). All figures in minutes. From St. James-Roberts and Halil (1991).

interpretation is that the evening crying peak is perceived by mothers to consist mainly of low intensity, fretful or irritable behaviour, rather than highly intense crying. This finding also highlights the definitional issues raised earlier, since methods which do not include fussing are likely to produce lower estimates of overall crying at this age.

4. As well as these common age-related changes in crying amount and pattern, there are large individual differences between the amounts infants cry. Given that such differences are the primary focus for clinical concern, it is disappointing that, although such differences are universally recognised, few figures have emerged so far to document them more precisely. The exception is St. James-Roberts and Halil's (1991) study, which is limited by the instrument – the Crying Patterns Questionnaire (CPQ) – used. The CPQ asks mothers to summarise the amount of time their babies spent fussing and

Table 1.1 Prevalence rates for 'persistent infant crying' at different ages. All figures are percentages of cases (from St. James-Roberts and Halil, 1991).

Definitions of 'persistent crying'	Age groups (months)			
	1–3	4–6	7–9	10–12
1. 24 hour fuss/crying ⩾ 4 hours	14	5	9	4
2. 24 hour fuss/crying ⩾ 3 hours	29	9	11	7
3. Fuss/crying ⩾ 2 hours in any one period	28	8	10	6
4. Fuss/crying ⩾ 1 hour in any one period	54	21	27	17

crying in each period of the previous day (or week if a regular daily pattern exists), so that a degree of estimation is necessarily involved.

The community crying rate figures found using the CPQ are summarised in Table 1.1. The majority of infants cried for 30 minutes or less in any given period of the day at all ages. However, a sizeable minority cried for prolonged amounts of time, particularly in the first few months. For example, if 'persistent' crying is defined as three hours or more in 24 hours, 29 per cent of 1–3-month infants were identified as persistent criers, declining to 7–11 per cent in months 4–12. As might be expected, the majority of such crying, particularly in the first three months, occurred in the evenings. That these figures are not too wide of the mark is indicated by Barr et al.'s (1991c) re-examination of the crying figures in Hunziker and Barr's (1986) diary measures of a normative control sample, 36 per cent of whom cried for three or more hours per day at six weeks of age. In Finland, 14 per cent of infants under three months were found to cry for three or more hours per day (Michelsson et al., 1990). As mentioned earlier, it is unclear whether this somewhat lower rate reflects cultural or methodological considerations.

5. For the most part, the studies to date have found little or no effect of infant sex or birth order on crying amount or pattern (St. James-Roberts and Halil, 1991). This conclusion must remain guarded since some earlier studies found higher amounts of fussing in boys (Moss, 1967). However, even where found, the differences are of a small magnitude, so that it does not appear that infant sex or birth order account substantially for persistent infant crying.

Measures of the impact of infant crying

As well as mothers' observations of infant crying, it is possible to assess the effects of the crying, both on the mothers and, via referral, on the health services and community. The distinction between crying and its impact is an important one, since not all parents will be distressed by – or seek help because of – infant crying. For instance, the Northamptonshire study found that mothers of firstborns were particularly likely to seek referral for excessive crying, presumably because inexperience raised their level of concern (St. James-Roberts and Halil, 1991). Other studies, too, have drawn attention to discrepancies between measures of crying and measures of whether it is a problem for parents (Danielsson and Hwang, 1985; Taubman, 1988). It seems likely that the psychological characteristics of parents, the amount of information they have about crying, non-crying aspects of infant behaviour (e.g. whether baby appears 'sick'), household arrangements and the availability of social support will all influence how parents respond to crying. Similarly, variations in the availability of primary healthcare in different localities will influence the rates of health-service referral which occur.

One reason for distinguishing crying from its impact is that clinical studies – that is, where parents have sought help from a health-service professional – are necessarily impact based. As a result, studies based on clinical samples may provide unrepresentative information about crying. A second reason is that crying impact measures are important in their own right, in assessing the 'cost' of infant crying for the community. For instance, measures of the amount of professional time devoted to crying problems may be used in auditing the health services. Since interventions aimed at infant crying should ideally reduce its effects on parents and others, impact measures can also be used to quantify the relative success of different treatments. At present, the range of impact measures available is limited so that, for example, we know little about the effects of crying on family members other than mothers. Ames (1989) has reported that fathers generally distance themselves from their babies' crying, so that their sleeping is less affected and they show less fatigue and depression. However, other family members and friends, as well as voluntary charitable organisations, provide support and more needs to be known about these provisions.

The two measures of crying impact – rates of associated maternal distress and of health-service referral – obtained in the Northamptonshire study are shown in Table 1.2. Two points are worth underscoring. First, the figures parallel the findings reported above, in that the major portion of maternal concern and referral coincides with the infant crying peaks. This implies both that maternal concerns are a direct reflection of infant crying levels and that phenomena occurring in infants generally in the early months underlie many

Table 1.2 Rates of maternal distress and referral to professionals because of persistent infant crying (from St. James-Roberts, 1991).

	Age groups (months) $N = 100$			
	1–3	4–6	7–9	10–12
Number of mothers upset by crying in the last week	20	7	13	13
Professional help sought recently	11	3	4	3

cases of referral. Second, in relation to Table 1.1, the Table 1.2 figures show, as expected, that not all mothers who reported high infant crying levels were disturbed by this. None the less, such concern was common, so that 21 per cent of the Northamptonshire and 15 per cent of London mothers sought referral at some point in the first three months. Unfortunately, no comparable figures from other studies are available. However, figures for infant 'colic' provide some basis for comparison, since referral for persistent crying is at the heart of this syndrome (see Chapter 2 for a fuller account of colic). On this basis, Rubin and Prendergast's (1984) rate of 26 per cent obtained by screening Norfolk mothers for colic in their infants is of the same order of magnitude as the figure found here.

In Finland, where monthly checkups are routine, Michelson *et al.* (1990) none the less found that 9 per cent of mothers wanted additional help for infant crying.

Crying in clinically referred infants

As the preceding figures show, western mothers refer a substantial minority of infants to health professionals because of infant crying they judge to be excessive. Given that the mothers may often know little about infant crying levels generally, an important question is whether the referred infants' crying differs from that in the general community.

Figure 1.3 shows maternal Crying Patterns Questionnaire measures for the Northamptonshire infants referred for excessive crying, compared with the

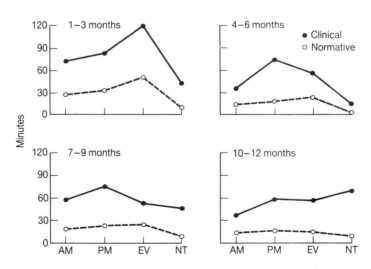

Figure 1.3 Mean crying minutes in the four age periods. From St. James-Roberts and Halil (1991).

Table 1.3 Maternal diary versus audiotape measures of the number of minutes of crying in referred and normative infants (from St. James-Roberts *et al.*, 1993).

	Referred infants ($N = 16$)		Normative infants ($N = 16$)	
	Diary mean (SD)	Audio-recording mean (SD)	Diary mean (SD)	Audio-recording mean (SD)
Morning (6 am–noon	38	48	27	25
Afternoon (noon–6 pm)	68	83	42	57
Evening (6 pm–mdnight)	75	79	46	49
Night (midnight–6 am)	16	20	21	18
24 hour total	197	230	136	149

equivalent measures in the general community. Table 1.3 shows comparable figures for a subset of the London infants who were tape-recorded. The referred infants in each case were gaining weight normally and none had a known organic disturbance. As Fig. 1.3 indicates, the amount of crying reported for the referred infants was approximately twice the average community level. The diary and tape-recorded figures (Table 1.3) show a similar but somewhat smaller difference partly due, perhaps, to exaggeration inherent in the questionnaire measures used in the Northants study. Also evident is that the referred infants showed the same crying patterns – including both time-of-day and developmental peaks – as the community infants. In more detailed analyses, St. James-Roberts and Halil (1991) found that 24 of 37 referred 1–3-month infants showed an evening crying peak, while night-time crying was a feature of referred 9–12 month olds. Crying in one period of the day was not sufficient, however, to account for the infants' high overall crying levels: the referred infants cried above mean community levels in several different periods of the day. A noteworthy finding from this study is that firstborns were particularly likely to be referred for excessive crying, although, as indicated earlier, there were no birth-order differences in crying amount or pattern. As well as highlighting the unrepresentativeness of clinically referred samples, this finding supports the important conclusion that maternal inexperience is associated with referral, but is not a major factor underlying persistent infant crying.

The finding that referred infants cry pervasively – in several different periods, rather than at one time of day – has prompted a recent examination of the *intensity* of referred infants' crying (St. James-Roberts *et al.*, 1991). It is possible that, as well as the amount and pattern, the intensity of crying is a factor underlying parental concern and referral. This analysis was also prompted by the finding, noted earlier, that the evening crying peak consists

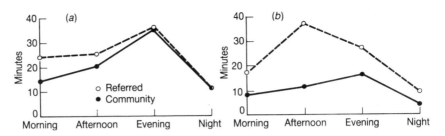

Figure 1.4 Fuss vs cry in community and referred infants. (a) Fussing at six weeks, (b) crying at six weeks.

predominantly of fretful, rather than intense, crying. An important proviso is that crying intensity was assessed by the poorly defined distinction between fussing and crying, while the analysis was based on maternal diary reports. The results are therefore best interpreted as evidence of whether referring mothers perceive their infants' crying to be relatively intense. The findings (Fig. 1.4) show that this is the case: both referred and normal–community six-week infants showed an evening fussing peak and this did not differ between the groups. In contrast, the referred infants were characterised by sustained crying, rather than fussing, at several times of the day. Although these findings must be regarded as provisional, they are consistent both with the clinical literature and with studies from other groups. Thus infants referred for crying have frequently been described as 'paroxysmal' or 'intense' in their crying (Wessel *et al.*, 1954; Lothe and Lindberg, 1989). Using objective, spectrographic analysis both Lester *et al.* (1992) and Zeskind and Barr (1992) have identified atypical pitch or other acoustic features in the cries of a subset of infants referred for persistent crying. It seems probable that such qualitative features are a part of the reason for parental perceptions and concerns.

The stability and outcome of infant crying

Although it has no precise meaning, the commonly used phrase 'a crying baby' carries the implication that particular infants both cry more than average and continue to do so in a relatively stable way. Whether, in fact, infants who cry persistently at one age show disturbances at older ages is a question of both practical and theoretical interest. For theoretical purposes, evidence of continuity will be consistent with explanations of behaviour problems which attribute these to constitutional traits in infants or to stable parent–infant interactions. For practical purposes, it is important to know whether, on the contrary, infants 'grow out of' their crying, as is often assumed. If so, it is a matter for debate whether this is a reason for deferring treatment (see Chapter

3). However, there seems little doubt that evidence of protracted disturbances will increase clinical concern about persistent infant crying. An important point is that, since infants' behaviour repertoires become more sophisticated as they grow older, stability in crying itself is not necessarily anticipated. Rather, the expectation is that stable crying in the early months will give way to disturbances in other areas of behaviour as the infants develop.

Although there are around fifteen studies of the stability and outcome of crying, the findings have to be interpreted with particular care. As well as the definitional caveats already noted, small sample sizes and further depletion with age are a feature of this area, so that it is hard to be confident about the representativeness of findings. An additional problem is that many of the studies have focused on the daylight hours, so that evening and night-time crying, which are important for parents and may contribute to stability, have been overlooked. As before, these considerations will be taken into account, so far as possible, in interpreting the studies' findings.

For the most part, studies of crying and irritability during the newborn period – the first few days after birth – indicate that day-to-day variability is the most striking feature of such behaviour at this age (Sameroff, 1978; St. James-Roberts and Wolke, 1988, 1989). Presumably, recovery from the birth process and adjustment to the postnatal environment are substantial influences for both infant and parents. One noteworthy exception is Korner *et al.*'s (1981) study, which found correlations of 0.36 to 0.80 in amounts of daytime crying across the first three postnatal days. Of these correlations, the highest (0.80) was obtained from just 14 infants, so that the day 1–2 correlation of 0.36, obtained from 44 infants, may be more typical. A feature of this study is that daytime crying was recorded by an automated apparatus while the infants were on four-hour feeding schedules in a hospital nursery. It is possible that such a standard regime increases the stability of individual differences in crying: an interpretation which is reinforced by Korner *et al.*'s finding that night-time crying, when the infants were fed on demand by their mothers, was not stable from day to day. Overall, it seems fair to conclude that individual stability in newborn crying, particularly under naturalistic circumstances, is of a low order.

Beyond the newborn period, moderate stabilities within the first 3–4 months have been found by the majority of studies (the exception being Bell and Ainsworth (1972), who found no stability within this period). Both Hubbard and van IJzendoorn (1991) and Isabella *et al.* (1985) found stability of 0.4–0.5 in overall fuss and crying, while Moss (1967) and Roe (1975) reported significant stabilities for fussing (around 0.4), while crying was unstable. Using the London maternal diary data set our own finding is that moderate correlations exist in both fuss and crying between weeks 2, 6 and 12. More specifically, babies who are among the top 20 per cent in amount of crying at 2 weeks are five times more likely than other infants to be in the top 20 per cent at 6 weeks, with a similar ratio between weeks 6 and 12 and a somewhat lower one between weeks 2 and 12. Consistent with Moss (1967) and Roe (1975), fussing is more stable than crying, so that high fussers at 6 weeks are eleven times more likely than the remaining infants to be high fussers at 12 weeks (St. James-Roberts and Plewis, 1992).

After three months of age, the figures already reported show that infants generally reduce the amount they cry by a substantial amount. Bearing this in mind, the question is whether high and low criers retain their relative status. The answer is that most studies have shown moderate correlations over periods of a few months in the middle or second half of the first year. The exceptions are Bell and Ainsworth (1972) and Hubbard and van IJzendoorn (1991), who found no significant correlations between the second and third quarters of the first year. However, Bell and Ainsworth (1972) reported significant, moderate crying correlations (0.4) between the third and fourth quarters, as did Snow et al. (1980). Low to moderate correlations have also been found between three and nine months (Fish and Crockenberg, 1981; Isabella et al., 1985), between six and thirteen months (Pettit and Bates, 1984; Roe, 1975) and between four, nine and fourteen months (Kagan and Snidman, 1991).

Since both crying and its impact are at their maximum in the first three postnatal months, the issue of most obvious clinical relevance is whether crying within the first quarter-year predicts longer-term problems, that is, disturbances towards the end of the first year and at older ages. The balance of the findings indicate low levels of predictability over this longer timescale. Hence, Hubbard and van IJzendoorn (1991), Isabella et al. (1985) and Snow et al. (1980) found no significant stabilities from the early weeks to 9–12 months of age. Matheny et al. (1985) reported a significant but low correlation (0.27) between newborn and nine-month irritability, while Fish and Crockenberg found no predictability from newborn fussiness, but significant stabilities in fussing between one, three and nine months. In the London diary data set we found no significant predictability for crying. As in the first two to three months, fussing is somewhat more stable, so that infants who are in the top 20 per cent for fussing at six weeks are six times as likely as other infants to be high fussers at nine months (St. James-Roberts and Plewis, 1992). As indicated earlier, part of the reason for this generally low level of predictability may be that infant characteristics have behaviour outlets other than crying at an older age. Taking this into account, the predictability of early crying becomes somewhat more reliable. Bernal (1973), for instance, reported that the group of infants who cried most in the newborn period was distinguished by sleeping problems at fourteen months, although the strength of this relationship was not reported. Likewise, other studies have reported early infant irritability to be moderately predictive of poor mother–infant interactions and attachment relationships at 12–18 months of age (Belsky et al., 1984; Crockenberg, 1981; Maccoby et al., 1984; van den Boom, 1988). In a recent study following infants with early crying problems to $3\frac{1}{2}$ years, Forsyth and

Canny (1991) reported a raised level of maternal perceptions of infant behaviour problems and vulnerabilities at this later age.

Taken as a whole, the implication of these findings is that infant crying, in particular, is not highly stable over the first year. Although infants are moderately consistent in the amounts they cry over periods of a few months, their relative crying levels are generally unstable over longer periods of time. In conjunction with the evidence that crying levels generally diminish after three months of age, these findings support the clinical maxim that infants generally 'grow out of' their crying. For parents, this is obviously an encouraging conclusion. None the less, the findings also indicate that infant fussing or irritability may be rather more stable than crying, while a minority of high criers continue to cry or to have other behaviour problems at older ages. Although this does not seem to be common, the dearth of longitudinal data means that it is impossible, at present, to estimate more exactly how often this happens, or to predict the cases where it is particularly likely to occur.

Studies in non-western communities

A limitation of the studies reported so far is that they all stem from western communities, which are relatively uniform in their approach to care. Findings from communities with alternative approaches are of especial significance, since they provide a test of the universality – or otherwise – of western infants' crying. For example, a finding of equivalent crying patterns, in spite of different care, would strongly indicate that the patterns are linked to maturational and developmental processes common to infants. A cross-cultural data-base will also address the vexed question of how much it is 'natural' for babies to cry. While this question is fraught with theoretical assumptions, evidence that western babies cry substantially more than those in other cultures might support the need to re-examine western practices of babycare.

Although there are anecdotal reports that infants in communities which employ frequent demand feeding and body contact cry less than western infants (Mead, 1935; Brazelton *et al.*, 1969), the most striking feature of the cross-cultural research literature is the lack of systematic studies. Only one detailed and scientifically robust study appears to have been published to date: that of Barr *et al.* (1991b), which stems from Konner's extensive observations of !Kung San infants in the Kalahari desert between 1969 and 1971. A strength of this study is that Konner's observations are known to be reliable, so that they can be interpreted as objective measures of infant crying. In addition, the study provides direct evidence that the !Kung San employ patterns of care which are untypical in the west. For instance, the infants were held or carried during 80 per cent of the daytime, while 92 per cent of infant frets or cries were responded to within fifteen seconds, usually with breast-feeding, which occurred on average four times each hour (Barr *et al.*, 1991b). A limitation is that, because Konner observed for short periods dispersed randomly over the daylight hours, time of day effects cannot be detected.

The study's main finding was a significant developmental crying 'peak', similar to that found in western studies, at about three months of age. Although this is slightly older than the peak crying age in the west, the study's methods leave it unclear whether this is a real age difference (Barr *et al.*, 1991b). This evidence of the universality of the infant crying peak was interpreted as indicative of a maturational or developmental process which occurs among infants generally at around this age (Barr *et al.*, 1991b). A second finding was that, compared with western infants, !Kung San infants cried as often, but for much shorter periods, than western infants. That is, their distressed behaviour consisted predominantly of short periods of fretful behaviour, rather than sustained crying bouts. As a result, the amount of crying per daylight hour (3.7 minutes) was much less than found in Dutch infants (7.2 minutes per hour) by Hubbard and van IJzendoorn (1987). On the face of it, this suggests that the total amount of !Kung San infants' crying may be substantially less than that of western infants. As Barr *et al.* (1991b) point out, however, this conclusion would be premature. One consideration, emphasised here, is that differences in how crying is defined and measured can lead to large differences in how much crying is reported, so that the same methods need to be used in two cultures in order to assess differences of crying amount. A second problem, as Barr *et al.* (1991b) note, is the lack of evening and night-time crying data for !Kung infants. Since there is other evidence that frequent breast-feeding is associated with more frequent waking and shorter sleep—wake cycles, it is possible that !Kung San infants cry as much as western infants, but with a more even distribution over day and night-time.

Summary and conclusions

1. Infant crying shows clear age and time-of-day crying peaks. In particular, raised crying levels within the first three months, particularly in the evenings, are common among western infants. At this age, the average daily crying total among western infants generally – around two hours per day – is substantial and evening crying makes up about 40 per cent of its total. Persistent infant crying, arbitrarily defined as three or more hours of fuss and crying per 24 hours, is also common at this age, being reported in around a quarter of western infants.

2. Both the daily total and the evening clustering of crying diminish markedly after three months of age. At around nine months, there is evidence of an increased prevalence of night-time crying. However, this is a rarer phenomenon and appears to be characteristic, particularly, of infants who fuss

and cry generally at that age. Conceivably, it heralds the onset of sleeping problems which are common in the second year (see Chapter 9).

3. The early infant crying peak in the general community underlies maternal distress and reports of crying as a problem. Such concerns are common, occurring in around 20 per cent of mothers in the United Kingdom. The referred infants show the same crying features as in the community, but cry substantially more than average. These findings suggest that referred infants may make up the extreme end of the normal distribution for crying. However, the referred infants' crying is distinguished: (1) by its pattern, in that the infants cry a lot in several different periods of the day; and (2) by its intensity, in that both clinical and research studies have identified intense crying as a feature of some referred infants. It seems likely that factors above and beyond those occurring in infants generally are involved in some referred cases, so that two or more subgroups of persistent crying may exist.

4. Since crying is a feature of feeding and sleeping problems, it is worth emphasising the degree to which persistent crying exists as an independent phenomenon in its own right. Compared with sleeping problems, the peak age for crying and crying problems is younger (the first three months of life, rather than the second year) and the daily distribution is different (with early crying occurring predominantly in the evening and afternoon, rather than at night). As other chapters in this book highlight, there is a closer developmental relationship with feeding problems. However, crying is only one result of feeding problems, while it is unclear how disturbances of feeding can account for the clustering of crying in a particular period of the day.

5. Although persistent crying is at the heart of parents' requests to professionals for help with excessive infant crying, it does not fully account for such requests. The available evidence suggests that crying features such as pattern and intensity, as well as amount, are involved. In addition, infant and parental features beyond actual crying are implicated. For some parents, irritable hard-to-soothe behaviour appears to be important (Barr *et al.*, 1988; St. James-Roberts, 1992b), so that measurements which distinguish such interactive behaviours from crying generally are needed. Likewise, parental perceptions that an infant is sick, variations in parental tolerance, maternal and family characteristics, and the absence of social support, may also be factors in referral.

Taken as a whole, these considerations emphasise the need to distinguish between crying and its social and clinical impact and highlight the dearth of research into crying as a social phenomenon. In particular, given the commonness and cost of infant crying as a primary health problem, the lack of routine community health-service provisions for managing the crying and supporting parents is striking.

6. Infant crying is not highly stable over the first year and this may be one reason for the current lack of provision. Predictability over periods of a few months is, however, moderate, so that some parents are exposed to substantial

levels of crying for several months at a time. The finding that most infants 'grow out of' their crying is a reassuring one for parents and practitioners alike. None the less, a minority of infants show a picture of protracted behaviour disturbances which extends beyond the first year. At present, it is not possible to predict these cases and more needs to be known about the factors responsible for the continuities.

References

Ames, E.W. (1989), 'The relation of infants' crying and sleep to their parents' sleep, moods and marital adjustment', Presented at the Third International Workshop in Infant Cry Research, Espoo, Finland, 13–18 July.

Barr, R.G. (1990), 'The normal crying curve: what do we really know?', *Developmental Medicine and Child Neurology*, 32, pp. 356–62.

Barr, R.G. and Desilets, J. (1992), 'The normal crying curve: hoops and hurdles', in B. Lester, J. Newman and F. Pederson (eds), *Biological and Social Aspects of Infant Crying* (New York: Plenum), in press.

Barr, R.G., Desilets, J. and Rotman, A. (1991a), 'Parsing the normal crying curve: is it really the evening fussing curve?', Presented at the 1991 Biennial Meeting of the Society of Research in Child Development, Seattle, 18–20 April.

Barr, R.G., Konner, N., Bakeman, R. and Adamson, L. (1991b), 'Crying in !Kung San infants: a test of the cultural specificity hypothesis', *Developmental Medicine and Child Neurology*, 33, pp. 601–10.

Barr, R.G., Kramer, M.S., Boisjoly, C., McVey-White, L. and Pless, I.B. (1988), 'Parental diary of infant cry and fuss behaviour', *Archives of Disease in Childhood*, 63, pp. 380–7.

Barr, R.G., McMullen, S.J., Spiess, H., Leduc, D.G., Yarenko, J., Barfield, R., Francoeur, T.E. and Hunziker, U. (1991c), 'Carrying as colic "therapy": a randomised controlled trial', *Pediatrics*, 87, pp. 623–30.

Bell, S.M. and Ainsworth, M.D.S. (1972), 'Infant crying and maternal responsiveness', *Child Development*, 43, pp. 1171–90.

Belsky, J., Rovine, M. and Taylor, D.G. (1984), 'The Pennsylvania infant and family development project III: the origins of individual differences in infant–mother attachment: maternal and infant contributions', *Child Developmentr*, 55, pp. 718–28.

Bernal, J.F. (1972), 'Crying during the first 10 days of life and maternal responses', *Developmental Medicine and Child Neurology*, 14, pp. 362–72.

Bernal, J.F. (1973), 'Night waking in infants during the first 14 months', *Developmental Medicine and Child Neurology*, 15, pp. 760–9.

Brazelton, T.B. (1962), 'Crying in infancy', *Pediatrics*, 29, pp. 579–88.

Brazelton, T.B., Robey, J.S. and Collier, G.A. (1969), 'Infant development in the Zinacanteco Indians of Southern Mexico', *Pediatrics*, 44, pp. 274–90.

Crockenberg, S. (1981), 'Infant irritability, mother responsiveness and social support influences on the security of infant-mother attachment', *Child Development*, 52, pp. 857–65.

Danielsson, B. and Hwang, C.P. (1985), 'Treatment of infantile colic with surface active substance (simethicone)', *Acta Paediatrica Scandinavica*, 74, pp. 446–50.

Fish, M. and Crockenberg, S. (1981), 'Correlates and antecedents of 9-month infant behaviour and mother–infant interaction', *Infant Behavior and Development*, 4, pp. 69–81.

Forsyth, B.W.C. and Canny, P.F. (1991), 'Perceptions of vulnerability $3\frac{1}{2}$ years after problems of feeding and crying behavior in early infancy', *Pediatrics*, 88, pp. 757–63.

Forsyth, B.W.C., Leventhal, J.M. and McCarthy, P.L. (1985), 'Mothers' perceptions of problems of feeding and crying behaviors. A prospective study', *American Journal of Disease in Childhood*, 139, pp. 269–72.

Frodi, A.M. (1981), 'Contribution of infant characteristics to child abuse', *American Journal of Mental Deficiency*, 85, pp. 341–9.

Frodi, A.M. (1985), 'When empathy fails: aversive infant crying and child abuse', in B.M. Lester and C.F.K. Boukydis (eds), *Infant crying: Theoretical and research perspectives* (New York: Plenum), pp. 263–78.

Hopkins, B. and van Wulfften-Palthe, T. (1987), 'The development of the crying state during early infancy', *Developmental Psychobiology*, 20, pp. 165–75.

Hubbard, F.O.A. and van IJzendoorn, M.H. (1987). 'Maternal unresponsiveness and infant crying: a critical replication of the Bell and Ainsworth study', in L.W.C. Tavecchio and M.H. van IJzendoorn (eds), *Attachment in Social Networks* (Amsterdam: Elsevier), pp. 339–75.

Hubbard, F.O.A. and van IJzendoorn, M.H. (1991), 'Maternal unresponsiveness and infant crying across the first 9 months: a naturalistic longitudinal study', *Infant Behavior and Development*, 14, pp. 299–312.

Hunziker, U.A. and Barr, R.G. (1986), 'Increased carrying reduces infant crying: a randomized control trial', *Pediatrics*, 77, pp. 641–8.

Isabella, R.A., Ward, M.J. and Belsky, J. (1985), 'Convergence of multiple sources of information on infant individuality: neonatal behavior, infant behavior, and temperament reports', *Infant Behavior and Development*, 8, pp. 283–91.

Kagan, J. and Snidman, N. (1991), 'Infant predictors of inhibited and uninhibited profiles', *Psychological Science*, 2, pp. 40–4.

Korner, A.F., Hutchinson, C.A., Koperski, J.A., Kraemer, H.C. and Schneider, P.A. (1981), 'Stability of individual differences of neonatal motor and crying patterns', *Child Development*, 52, pp. 83–90.

Lester, B.M., Boukydis, C.F.Z., Garcia-Coll, C., Hole, W.T. and Peucker, M. (1992), 'Infantile colic: acoustic cry characteristics, maternal perception of cry, and temperament', *Infant Behavior and Development*, 15, pp. 15–26.

Lieberman, P. (1985), 'The physiology of cry and speech in relation to linguistic behaviour', in B.M. Lester and C.F.Z. Boukydis (eds), *Infant Crying: Theoretical and research perspectives* (New York: Plenum).

Lothe, L. and Lindberg, T. (1989), 'Cow's milk whey protein elicits symptoms of infantile colic in colicky formula-fed infants: a double blind crossover study', *Pediatrics*, 83, pp. 262–6.

Maccoby, E.E., Snow, M.E. and Jacklin, C.N. (1984), 'Children's dispositions and mother–child interaction at 12 and 18 months: a short-term longitudinal study', *Developmental Psychology*, 20, pp. 459–72.

Matheny, A.P., Riese, M.L. and Wilson, R.S. (1985), 'Rudiments of infant temperament: newborn to nine months', *Developmental Psychology*, 21, pp. 486–94.

Mead, M. (1935), *Sex and Temperament in Three Primitive Societies* (London: Routledge & Kegan Paul).

Michelson, K., Rinne, A. and Paajen, S. (1990), 'Crying, feeding and sleeping patterns in 1 to 12 month-old-infants', *Child: Care, Health and Development*, 26, pp. 99–111.

Moss, H.A. (1967), 'Sex, age and state as determinates of mother–infant interaction', *Merrill-Palmer Quarterly*, **13**, pp. 19–36.

Pettit, G.S. and Bates, J.E. (1984), 'Continuity of individual differences in the mother–infant relationship from six to thirteen months', *Child Development*, **55**, 729–39.

Prechtl, H.F.R. (1974), 'The behavioural states of the newborn: a review', *Brain Research*, **76**, pp. 185–202.

Roe, K.V. (1975), 'Amount of infant vocalisation as a function of age: some cognitive implications', *Child Development*, **46**, pp. 936–41.

Rubin, S.P. and Prendergast, M. (1984), 'Infantile colic: incidence and treatment in a Norfolk community', *Child: Care, Health and Development*, **10**, pp. 219–26.

St. James-Roberts, I. (1991), 'Persistent infant crying', *Archives of Disease in Childhood*, **66**, pp. 653–5.

St. James-Roberts, I. (1992a), 'Managing infants who cry persistently', *British Medical Journal*, **304**, pp. 997–8.

St. James-Roberts, I. (1992b), 'Measuring infant crying and its social perception and impact', *Association for Child Psychology and Psychiatry Newsletter*, **14**, pp. 128–31.

St. James-Roberts, I., Bowyer, J. and Hurry, J. (1991), 'Delineating "problem" infant crying: findings in community and referred infants, using tape recordings, diaries and questionnaires', Presented at the 1991 Biennial Meeting of the Society for Research in Child Development, Seattle, 18–20 April.

St. James-Roberts, I., Bowyer, J. and Hurry, J. (1993), 'Crying and fussing in infants referred for excessive crying and in controls: audiotape versus diary measures', in preparation.

St. James-Roberts, I. and Halil, T. (1991), 'Infant crying patterns in the first year: normative and clinical findings', *Journal of Child Psychology and Psychiatry*, **32**, pp. 951–68.

St. James-Roberts, I. and Plewis, I. (1992), 'Infant behaviour problems: stabilities and links between problems in the first year', Presented at the Annual Conference of the British Psychological Society: Developmental Section, Edinburgh, 11–14 September.

St. James-Roberts, I. and Wolke, D. (1988), 'Convergences and discrepancies among mothers' and professionals' assessments of difficult neonatal behaviour', *Journal of Child Psychology and Psychiatry*, **29**, pp. 21–42.

St. James-Roberts, I. and Wolke, D. (1989), 'Do obstetric factors affect the mother's perception of her new-born's behaviour?', *British Journal of Developmental Psychology*, **7**, pp. 141–58.

Sameroff, A.J. (1978), 'Organisation and stability of newborn behavior: a commentary on the Brazelton Neonatal Behavioral Assessment Scale', *Monographs of the Society for Research in Child Development*, **43** (5–6), serial No. 177.

Snow, M.E., Jacklin, C.N. and Maccoby, E.E. (1980), 'Crying episodes and sleep–wakefulness transitions in the first 26 months of life', *Infant Behavior and Development*, **3**, pp. 387–94.

Taubman, B. (1988), 'Parental counselling compared with elimination of cow's milk or soy milk protein for the treatment of infant colic syndrome: a randomized trial', *Pediatrics*, **81**, pp. 756–61.

Thompson, R.A. and Lamb, M.E. (1983), 'Individual differences in dimensions of socioemotional development in infancy', in R. Plutchik and H. Kellerman (eds), *Emotion: Theory, research and experience*, vol. 2, (London: Academic), pp. 87–114.

van den Boom, D. (1988), 'Neonatal irritability and the development of attachment: observation and intervention', PhD Dissertation, University of Leiden, The Netherlands.

Wasz-Hockert, O., Michelsson, K. and Lind, J. (1985), 'Twenty-five years of Scandinavian cry research', in B.M. Lester and C.F.Z. Boukydis (eds), *Infant Crying: Theoretical and research perspectives* (New York: Plenum), pp. 349–54.

Wessel, M.A., Cobb, J.C., Jackson, E.B., Harris, G.S. and Detwiler, A.C. (1954), 'Paroxysmal fussing in infancy, sometimes called "colic"', *Pediatrics*, 14, pp. 421–35.

Wolff, P.H. (1987), *The Development of Behavioral States and the Expression of Emotions in Early Infancy* (Chicago: University of Chicago Press).

Zeskind, P.S. and Barr, R.G. (1992), 'Acoustic analysis of cries of infants with and without colic', Presented to the Conference on Human Development, Atlanta, GA, April.

Zeskind, P.S. and Lester, B.H. (1978), 'Acoustic features and auditory perceptions of the cries of newborns with prenatal and perinatal complications', *Child Development*, 49, pp. 580–9.

Zeskind, P.S., Sale, J., Maio, M.L., Huntington, L. and Weiseman, J.R. (1985), 'Adult perceptions of pain and hunger cries: a synchrony of arousal', *Child Development*, 56, pp. 549–54.

Chapter 2

Explanations of persistent infant crying

Ian St. James-Roberts, *University of London*

There is no shortage of explanations for persistent infant crying. Indeed, until quite recently conjecture and theorising about the causes of crying have run far in advance of the evidence available about crying itself. As Chapter 1 indicates, this picture has begun to change and basic information about crying in the general community and in infants referred for excessive crying has become available. We now know what there is to explain. As the previous chapter also illustrates, the situation is made more complex by the fact that it is parents, not infants, who seek referral to healthcare professionals for infant crying problems. The practical issue of 'crying problems' is therefore a social one and part of what needs to be explained is what leads some parents to view as problematic crying which other parents do not. Chapter 1 concludes that this social phenomenon probably reflects other infant variables as well as parental and community ones and emphasises the need for more detailed information on the factors involved.

Although it is important to understand crying as a social phenomenon, the evidence reviewed in Chapter 1 also makes clear that variations in the amount and other features of infant crying are central to the practical picture. It is the case: (1) that large individual differences in infant crying exist; (2) that a sizeable minority of infants cry for what seem to be substantial amounts of time; (3) that they remain relatively high criers for periods of several months; and (4) that infants referred for 'excessive crying' do, in fact, cry considerably more than average. This chapter's aim will therefore be to examine the main explanations advanced to account for these individual differences in crying. In each case, the approach adopted will be to outline the main features of the explanation, distinguish the predictions it makes, and consider how far these are compatible with the available evidence. It is not intended that a single explanation of persistent infant crying will result. Because the infant's behaviour repertoire is limited, crying serves as a 'final common pathway' for a variety of infant needs and disturbances. As a result, it seems likely that a number of factors contribute to variations in infant crying, so that the causes of crying in one infant will differ from those in another. Bearing this in mind, this chapter's overall goal will be to identify the most likely candidates and to outline a conceptual framework which will help to integrate research and practice in this area. It is acknowledged that crying may be due to a variety of illnesses. However, these are usually detectable by routine clinical practice (Poole, 1991; Valman, 1989), so that the focus will be on crying as described in Chapter 1 and for which there is no obvious explanation.

Although a considerable number of possible explanations for persistent crying exist, the main theories can be distinguished according to whether the crying is attributed to infant or environmental factors, and whether or not an organic disturbance is implicated. In particular, five main explanations can be identified: (1) colic; (2) neurological disorders; (3) temperament; (4) normal developmental processes; and (5) inadequate parental care and attachment.

Colic

As a previous review has noted (St. James-Roberts, 1991), there is no agreed definition for colic and the word has at least three distinct meanings. Arguably the most common usage is to refer to the amount and, to a lesser degree, intensity of infant crying. Wessel *et al.*'s (1954) widely used 'rule of threes', for example, defines colic as 'paroxysms of irritability, fussing, or crying lasting for a total of more than three hours a day and occurring on more than three days in any one week' (pp. 425–6). In this sense, the word colic is essentially a descriptive one and overlaps with the term 'persistent crying' used here. There is no particular reason for the choice of three or more hours a day as a cut-off. However, this criterion is emerging as an effective 'rule of thumb' for identifying infants who cry substantially more than average.

The second usage is to designate parental referral for problem crying. Barr *et al.* (1991a), for instance, define colic as 'crying seen as a problem by both mother and physician' (p. 624). This is a workable definition for clinical purposes but, as Chapter 1 points out, it refers to subjective factors in parents and clinicians as well as to infant variables.

The third and more specific use of the term 'colic' is an explanatory, rather than descriptive, one and is of most relevance here. As Carey (1984) has noted, the word colic derives from the Greek *Kolikos*, the adjective of *Kolon*, implying the existence of a gastrointestinal disturbance which causes discomfort or pain. This view of colic is widely held (Illingworth, 1985). It follows that two main kinds of evidence are needed to substantiate the existence of colic as an explanation for crying. First, it is necessary to show that the crying is 'painful' and part of a syndrome of pain-related behaviour more generally. Second, an explanation is needed for why a substantial minority of normal infants should experience gastrointestinal disorders, while others do not. More specifically, the following findings are needed to substantiate a colic explanation of persistent crying:

1. Compared to crying generally, colic crying should be of a high intensity and show the acoustic qualities of 'pain crying'.
2. The crying should be reliably accompanied by other behaviours indicative of pain, e.g. writhing, facial grimaces and muscular hypertonia.
3. The crying should be inconsolable, that is, persistent in spite of routine caregiver interventions (picking up/cuddling, carrying, feeding) and typified by sustained crying periods or 'bouts'.
4. Since the crying is presumed to be digestion related, the times of crying periods should be synchronised to the times of feeds.
5. Evidence of abnormal gastrointestinal function is needed, together with an explanation of why this should occur. Since colic affects only a minority of infants and is traditionally defined as self-limiting to the first three months, these properties need to be accounted for as well.

As previous reviews have shown (Illingworth, 1985; Barr, 1989), the view that crying is due to gastrointestinal disturbance has produced a substantial literature, but very little evidence that this is the case. For example, no abnormalities of intestinal mobility or function, or of breath hydrogen production – which would be indicative of lactose or other digestive deficiencies – have been reliably found in infants diagnosed as 'colicky' because of their crying (Barr *et al.*, 1991c; Hyams *et al.*, 1989). A related problem is that some symptoms of gastric disturbance may result from (rather than cause) extended periods of crying.

In view of this dearth of direct supportive evidence, the mainstay of the colic hypothesis, until recently, has been the finding that the anticholinergic drug dicyclomine hydrochloride led to reduced crying in many cases (see Chapter 3). It is possible that the mechanism of this drug's action involved the intestinal musculature. However, since complications such as drowsiness and respiratory difficulties were reported (and led the manufacturer to recommend against dicyclomine's use with infants) it is also possible that the drug's therapeutic effect was on the nervous system rather than on digestive functions.

Although this background of poor support for colic as a cause of crying remains, several recent studies have provided evidence which is at least partly consistent with the predictions outlined above. In particular, two independent studies have provided evidence which is suggestive of painful behaviour in a subgroup of infants selected for persistent crying. In Lester *et al.*'s (1992) case, 16 of 160 infants participating in a longitudinal study were selected because (1) they were reported to meet Wessel *et al.*'s (1954) 'rule of threes' definition of persistent crying; (2) the crying had a 'paroxysmal onset'; (3) they were inconsolable and hypertonic; and (4) they were reported to have an aversive high-pitched cry. Subsequent computer analyses showed that these infants' cries were indeed abnormal in pitch and acoustically 'turbulent' during mildly stressful procedures, compared with controls. In the second study, Zeskind and Barr (1992), again using Wessel *et al.*'s (1954) criterion to select infants, found atypical acoustic features in the cries of such infants *after*, but *not before*, their dinner. In further analyses, Barr *et al.* (1991b) found these infants to differ from controls in their facial expressions *before*, but *not after*, feeds. Both the reason for this before:after feed variability and some other technical issues need to be resolved (for instance, Zeskind and Barr (1992) did not find the difference in fundamental frequency identified by Lester *et al.* (1992)). None the less (and leaving aside the thorny issue of how to prove the existence of pain in infants), these studies provide the first evidence that at least some infants who cry a lot are displaying atypical cries and other behaviours suggestive of pain. For clinical purposes, an important question is how many infants are involved. Unfortunately, the methods used by these studies do not allow this to be accurately determined. In Lester *et al.*'s study, 10 per cent of infants were chosen but the initial longitudinal cohort was also especially selected. In Barr *et al.*'s analyses, the initial group of referred infants was broken down into about a third who met Wessel *et al.*'s (1954) definition – and who were distinguishable by their cries and facial expressions – and about two thirds who did not meet Wessel *et al.*'s definition – who did not differ from normal controls on acoustic or facial-expression analyses. If this picture is representative, it suggests that pain as a possible cause of crying is detectable in a minority of referred infants.

Although the existence of pain is one prerequisite of a colic interpretation of crying, it is also necessary to provide evidence of a gastrointestinal basis for pain. Barr and colleagues' finding of a link between crying and feed-times, although not straightforward, is along these lines. Several recent studies – reviewed more extensively by Wolke in Chapter 3 – have provided more direct evidence of a possible gastrointestinal disturbance, involving cow's milk intolerance, in some cases. In addition, Lothe *et al.* (1990) have identified a possible mechanism, involving gut immaturity or deficits in the peptide hormone motilin. As with pain, the chief issue in understanding the contribution of gastrointestinal disturbance to crying, at least from a clinical point of view, is how commonly this occurs. It is again difficult to arrive at a precise figure. Lothe and Lindberg (1989) state that the infants in their study comprised 10 per cent of the approximately 17 per cent of infants diagnosed as having colic in Malmö, that is, about 2 per cent of infants overall. If so, this suggests that cow's-milk-related gastrointestinal disorder accounts for a small subgroup of the overall number of infants who cry persistently and/or who are referred for persistent crying.

In sum, there is growing evidence for the existence of a small, but important, subgroup of infants whose crying is related to pain which, at least in some cases, has a gastrointestinal basis. The size of this 'true colic' group remains to be reliably determined, but it seems unlikely to account for crying in more than a small proportion of cases. At present, evidence is lacking as to why colic should affect some infants and not others, why it should affect crying most strongly in the evenings, and why it should be confined to the early months of infancy.

Central or autonomic nervous system disorder

Rather than gastrointestinal disturbance, infant crying or irritability may also be due to neurological disorders or disturbances. Such disorders may be mild and transitory or more severe and persistent, and may be either due to pregnancy and childbirth complications or be of unknown origins. The chief expected crying and associated features of infants with nervous system disorders are:

1. Crying which is abnormal in pitch or other qualitative features, but not predominantly pain crying.
2. Evidence of atypical central or autonomic nervous system functioning.
3. A raised prevalence of genetic anomalies, or of exposure to biological hazards, such as pregnancy and childbirth complications.

Although there is ample evidence that infants exposed to severe pre- and perinatal complications have high-pitched, qualitatively abnormal cries (Lester and Boukydis, 1985; Huntingdon *et al.*, 1990; Zeskind and Lester, 1978), there is much less evidence that such complications are associated with raised *amounts* of infant crying. In some instances, initial findings consistent with this hypothesis have not been replicated (Woodson *et al.*, 1979). In others, effects of pre- and peri-natal complications were detected during controlled newborn behaviour tests, but had little impact on behaviour in more naturalistic settings and were not perceived by mothers (St. James-Roberts and Wolke, 1988, 1989). One probable reason for such inconsistency, indicated in Chapter 1, is the high day-to-day variability which is particularly characteristic of newborn infants. A second is that although biological adversities may sometimes increase irritability, in other cases they may weaken and impair newborn functioning, leading to reduced crying and under-aroused, hypotonic, rather than hypertonic behaviour. A third consideration is that it is difficult, in practice, to separate the effects of pre- and perinatal complications from the consequences of other variables. To take one example, there is reliable evidence that anxious women have a raised level of obstetric complications (Holmes *et al.*, 1984). A finding of irritability in newborns exposed to such complications can therefore be explained equally well by the complications, by the newborns' genetic dispositions and by the effect of inadequate maternal postnatal care. Disentangling such influences requires considerable ingenuity and research expenditure and has so far not yielded to the resources available. Perhaps the most which can safely be concluded from the existing research is that severe pregnancy and childbirth hazards are related to the quality of infant crying and may well contribute to variations in amount, but that this remains to be established.

Putting the question of the origins of any neurological disorders to one side, it is the case that a number of research groups have recently provided evidence of a link between atypical autonomic nervous system functioning and crying in response to challenging conditions (DeGangi *et al.*, 1991; Fox, 1989; Kagan and Snidman, 1991; Lester *et al.*, 1992). In each case, the implication is that a subgroup of infants, perhaps 8 to 10 per cent, has difficulty in modulating their internal physiological state in response to arousing stimuli. Lester *et al.* (1990), in particular, sugggest that such infants lack self-regulatory capacities for soothing because of autonomic imbalance, that is, heightened sympathetic arousal combined with inadequate parasympathetic inhibitory control. This model is attractive, because excessive sympathetic excitation can account for increased gastric activity and for several other features of colic, as well as for infant irritability. It remains unclear, however, why colic in this case should show a decline after three months of age. Related to this, Lester *et al.* (1990) appear undecided as to whether the putative autonomic imbalance is evidence of a chronic disturbance, a reflection of normal individual difference, or an indication of a short-term maturational delay. In contrast, DeGangi *et al.* (1991) refer to 'Regulatory Disordered' infants and deliberately distinguish these from infants who show short-term colic or sleep disorders. These findings, then, leave it unclear whether autonomic reactivity is a disturbance which requires treatment, or a reflection of something more akin to temperament. The studies are, however, impressively consistent in their general finding that individual differences in autonomic reactivity can play a part in modulating infants' responses to stressful circumstances. An important next step is to link such reactivities to naturalistic crying behaviour. If such links can be shown, this approach appears promising both in accounting for variations in infants' susceptibility to crying and in providing assessments which enable vulnerable infants to be identified.

Temperament

The idea that some infants are difficult by nature owes its origins to the New York Longitudinal Study of temperament (NYLS: Thomas *et al.*, 1968; Thomas and Chess, 1977). Starting in the first few months of infancy, this landmark study found approximately 10 per cent of some 140 infants they followed to be especially intense, irregular, negative, withdrawing and

unadaptable: a cluster of behaviours which was labelled 'difficult temperament'. As these infants grew older, they were found to be particularly at risk
for the development of behavioural and psychiatric problems.

Like the concept of colic, the general notion of temperament is widely
accepted but hard to define in a precise and testable way, so that contemporary
temperament research includes a diversity of definitions and methodological
approaches (Goldsmith *et al.*, 1987). Compared with colic and cerebral
disturbance, temperament appears to refer to normal individual differences
between individuals (rather than to a disorder) and to constitutionally based
characteristics which are relatively stable over age. Hence, the following
predictions follow from a temperamental interpretation of crying:

1. The infants in question should show persistent and possibly intense, but
   qualitatively normal, crying. There should be average levels of pain crying
   and no particular clustering of crying with other pain-related behaviour.
2. Differences in the relative amounts infants cry should remain stable over
   age.
3. As the infants develop, there should be concurrent and predictive
   associations with other aspects of difficult temperament (withdrawal,
   intensity, unadaptability, etc.).
4. There should be no evidence of organic disturbance.
5. The crying should not be a direct result of parental care. That is, the
   infants' parents should show the normal range of approaches to care.

The view that there is a link between temperament and infant crying
remains popular, both among parents and researchers (Barr *et al.*, 1983; Bates,
1983; Crockenberg and Smith, 1982; Lester *et al.*, 1992; St. James-Roberts
and Wolke, 1988). Some writers appear to have applied the NYLS findings
directly to crying, for example by claiming that 10 per cent of infants are
'crybabies' (Gray, 1987), although, as Chapter 1 indicates, there is little basis
for this figure. Given that the NYLS findings are in danger of being
over-interpreted, it is important to establish that the NYLS itself provides no
direct evidence that difficult temperament underlies persistent crying. For one
thing, the stability and predictiveness found for 'difficult' behaviour emerged
only gradually in the NYLS, becoming significant only beyond two years of
age (Thomas *et al.*, 1968; Thomas and Chess, 1986). Indeed, Thomas *et al.*
(1982) have themselves stressed that difficult temperament and crying should
not be treated as synonymous.

Thomas *et al.*'s (1982) distinction between crying and difficult temperament is readily illustrated with reference to the Louisville study (Matheny *et
al.*, 1984, 1985; Matheny, 1986; Riese, 1987), which is arguably the most
extensive and methodologically sophisticated study in this area. Unlike the
NYLS, this study included objective assessments of temperament, as well as
parental measures, condensing the measures over methods and occasions to

produce a core dimension labelled 'irritability' which shared several of the NYLS elements of 'difficult behaviour'. To examine stability, this irritability dimension was used to predict an age-adjusted but analogous dimension (emotional tone) at older ages. The finding was that stability from the newborn period was patchy and of a low order, with correlations of 0.2 to 0.3 with 9-month, and 0.3 to 0.4 with 24-month temperament measures, but no significant correlations with the same measures at the in-between ages of 12 and 18 months (Riese, 1987). However, the across-age stabilities increased as the infants became older, reaching a moderate level between 12 and 18 months and a quite substantial level (0.7) between 18 and 24 months (Matheny, 1986). By comparing monozygotic with dizygotic twin pairs, Riese (1990) later reported no genetic contribution to newborn irritability and concluded that genetic influence increases with age.

Returning to Thomas *et al.*'s (1982) distinction betweeen crying and difficult temperament, the Louisville study findings have two main implications. The first is that the contribution of temperament to irritability in young infants is modest, but increases with age. This may seem counter-intuitive, given the traditional assumption that temperament provides the biological substrates onto which experience builds. However, this need not be the case if the first year of life is viewed as a period predominantly of physical growth and developmental transition, so that the neurophysiological substrates of mature behaviour have not yet developed (see the next section in this chapter). Moreover, it is consistent with other evidence on the behavioural, physiological and genetic aspects of temperament (Riese, 1990). Fox (1989), in particular, has found that heart-rate and vagal tone indices, which are viewed as the substrates of emotional responsivity, are unstable during the first half of the year, becoming increasingly stable thereafter.

The Louisville study's second implication is to highlight the distinction between irritability as a reflection of temperament and the phenomenon of persistent crying identified in Chapter 1. A feature both of the Louisville study and of others which have shown significant stability in early infancy is the use of standard, mildly stressful, procedures which elicit behaviour under controlled conditions (Kagan and Snidman, 1991; Worobey and Lewis, 1989; see also Chapter 1). In effect, the studies' finding is that of moderate consistency in infants' reactions to demanding social and physical stimuli, particularly in highly selected, 'extreme' groups of infants. On one hand, this finding is consistent with some of the findings from crying research, in that much of the behaviour mothers report is irritable, fretful behaviour requiring frequent and persistent interventions on the mothers' part (Chapter 1). On the other hand, it is hard to see how temperament seen in this way – that is, as a moderator of infant reactivity – can account for two of the main features of persistent infant crying: the clustering of crying at a particular time of the day and the age-related decline in crying which occurs among infants generally after three months. It seems more likely that the role of temperament is to amplify or modulate infant responses to other stresses, so that it is reflected, for instance, in a more pronounced time-of-day peak or in a relatively intense response to stressful stimulation which remains stable with age. Unfortunately, there are few direct studies of the relationship between temperament and crying, specifically, in naturalistic settings, and for the most part these have focused on concurrent relationships between crying and maternal ratings of temperament. Barr *et al.* (1991b) and Lester *et al.* (1992), for example, have both reported that infants who cry a great deal are rated as difficult by their mothers at the same age, a finding that is neither surprising nor persuasive evidence of a stable temperament. More convincingly, Barr *et al.* (1983) found that maternal ratings of temperament at two weeks predicted the duration of infant fuss and crying at six weeks. However, the proportion of variation in the six-week crying measures accounted for was minimal (7 per cent) and no objective evidence of the infants' temperamental characteristics was provided.

In sum, there is little basis in the available evidence for the conclusion that temperament provides an explanation for all or most of the features of persistent infant crying. It appears most likely that the role of temperament is to modulate infants' reactiveness to other, physical and social, demands. In particular, there is consistent and growing evidence that temperament may be expressed in infant irritability and that its contribution is initially small but increases with age. If confirmed, this conclusion has both practical and theoretical implications. From a research point of view, it suggests the need to distinguish irritability from crying more generally in future studies. For practical purposes, the finding that some infants react strongly to demanding circumstances may be helpful for parents, since knowledge that an infant has special needs can offset feelings of guilt and enable a more positive and flexible approach to infant care.

Normal maturational and developmental processes

In contrast to temperament's focus on stable differences between individuals, the focus here is on processes of change which are common to all children. Underlying this perspective is the view that infancy is first and foremost a period of major transition and adjustment. At the outset, the infant has to adapt to the postnatal environment and, during the next few months, to rapid changes in physiological, psychological and social capacities. Infant crying is attributed to the resulting disruptions and reorganisations of physiological systems. A further implication is that the neurophysiological and mental substrates underlying crying and other behaviour will change as infants develop. Compared to the other explanations of infant crying, this perspective makes the following predictions:

1. Crying should show marked variations with age and individual stability should be low.
2. Infants who cry a lot at any one age represent the extreme tip of the normal distribution. Their crying should be qualitatively normal and display the same features as that of other infants, differing only in degree.
3. The crying should coincide with periods of marked change in other areas of physiological, psychological or social development.
4. The causes of crying will vary as the infant's capabilities and needs develop. A distinction can therefore be drawn between causes at early and later ages and between the factors which initiate and which sustain crying.
5. There should be no evidence of organic pathology.
6. The crying should be largely independent of within- and between-culture variations of care.

The view that developmental reorganisations or 'shifts' are at the heart of persistent infant crying is a popular one (Barr, 1990; Emde *et al.*, 1976; Lester, 1985; St. James-Roberts, 1989). It draws substance from the finding amongst both psychologists and neurologists that major neurobehavioural transitions occur at around three and nine months of age. In particular, the period around three months sees the disappearance of a number of so-called 'primitive reflexes' and, by implication, the emergence of cortical regulatory control over the reflexive nervous systems responsible for behaviour up to that age (Lester, 1985; Prechtl, 1984). By twelve weeks, too, sleep–waking organisation has been transformed to show a diurnal cycle, with the majority of infants sleeping through the night (Parmelee and Stern, 1972). Changes occur in learning abilities, so that infants can inhibit crying more readily (Fisichelli *et al.*, 1974) and begin to anticipate caregiver behaviour (Gekoski *et al.*, 1983). At a social level, smiling becomes established and the infant becomes a more responsive interactive partner (Lamb, 1981). As the other chapters of this book indicate, this is also a time of change for feeding practices, with the peak age for abandoning breast-feeding occurring, at least in the United Kingdom, at around six weeks.

In broad terms, this view that persistent crying is due to the difficulties some infants have in making normal developmental transitions is an attractive one, partly because it suggests that infants who cry a great deal are developing normally and partly because it maps well onto several of the main features of persistent crying and referral identified in Chapter 1. In particular, the evidence of a common crying peak in the first three months, finding that many infants 'grow out of' their crying, and finding of a shift to night-time crying at around nine months, can all be accommodated within this framework. However, this explanation also leaves a great deal unresolved. One obvious shortcoming, given that all infants make such developmental shifts, is why some infants make them easily – without crying much – while others find them difficult and cry a great deal. Strictly speaking, a developmental explanation allows differences in the rate of development only (i.e. immaturity) to be advanced to explain persistent crying and it is unclear how they could do so. Individual difference factors, such as temperament, are therefore needed to explain why some infants find the transitions difficult. A second limitation is that it is not apparent why developmental processes should cause crying in the evening in particular. A third is that development fails to account for the finding of particularly intense crying among some referred infants. Lastly, this perspective is vague about the nature and direction of causation. For example, it is possible that crying is due to specific 'developmental problems', such as feeding and associated nutritional deficiencies, or that both crying and feeding problems are linked to a more general neurobehavioural reorganisation. If Loethe *et al.* (1990) are correct in attributing cow's milk intolerance to gastrointestinal immaturity, it is also possible to view colic as essentially a developmental phenomenon.

Given that the main point of a theoretical explanation is to enable specific predictions to be made, this vagueness is unhelpful. So far, only two attempts to refine this general approach into more specific proposals have been made. In one case, noting that the development of crying parallels the development of a diurnal sleep–waking cycle, Hurry *et al.* (1991) proposed that the early crying peak was a consequence of the daytime sleep reduction which occurs as sleep is shifted from day to night-time. This hypothesis was partly supported, in that high crying was found to be associated with relatively low levels of sleeping. However, it was not the case that infants who cried a lot were delayed in the age at which a diurnal sleep–wake cycle was established. Hence, this study provides no evidence that sleep reorganisation causes crying. The second model, attributing crying to inadequate development of the autonomic nervous system (Lester *et al.*, 1990) has been examined in the section on neurological disorders in this chapter. As indicated there, it is uncertain whether this explanation refers to maturational differences between infants, to chronic disturbances, or to normal individual differences. The model has the potential to account both for 'colicky' infant features and for crying, but it is at an early stage of refinement and awaits direct supportive evidence.

In short then, the developmental explanation currently provides a broad conceptual framework which seems able to account for several of the main features of persistent infant crying, but which requires refinement and is unlikely to provide a sufficient explanation. One other implication of this approach is, however, worth highlighting: the premise that the causes of crying will change with age. By general consensus, crying does change its function as infants get older, developing from an essentially reflexive, unlearned and asocial sign of distress and discomfort into a learned and differentiated behaviour which reflects the development of emotional abilities and modulates social interaction. As Lamb (1981) has pointed out, crying provides the growing infant with the opportunity to learn and develop expectations about the consequences of its behaviour and to acquire the rudiments of social and affectionate communication. Gustafson and Green (1991) provide further evidence of this process.

This conclusion that crying changes its function with age has important implications, in turn, for parental behaviour and for crying treatment studies. For parents, it follows from this developmental perspective that the optimum caregiving behaviour will vary as infants grow older. Initially, the reflexive nature of crying implies the need for a predominant strategy of responding to crying. As learning and social communicative abilities develop, however, a strategy of uncritical response will prevent the infant from learning differentiated social communicative skills and autonomous self-control, both of which are desirable in the longer term. At this later stage, then, it becomes important to 'read' the likely reason for the crying and to take more account of social learning principles. As noted below, there is evidence that many parents do gradually adopt an interpretative, wait-and-see response to some aspects of crying as social communication develops (Hubbard and van IJzendoorn, 1987, 1991; Wolff, 1987). For professionals seeking to treat infant crying, these developmental changes in crying's function are equally critical, since they imply the need for an increased focus on learning and social processes as infants develop. In addition, it is important to bear in mind the delay which has occurred between crying onset and referral, since the factors underlying and maintaining the crying may have changed in the interim period.

Inadequate parental care or attachments

Infant crying has often been blamed on deficiencies of parental care. One possibility is that inadequacies of feeding or of another type which produce organic impairments are to blame. Alternatively, the deficiencies may be attributed less to physiological than to unmet psychological needs. Bowlby (1982) proposed the existence of an intrinsic attachment system, whereby infant crying elicits proximity and stimulation from the caregiver. Prolonged crying is then attributed to parental failure to meet the infant's biological need for physical contact and affectionate, responsive care. More specifically, an attachment explanation for persistent crying makes the following predictions:

1. Prolonged crying should be associated with delayed parental response, frequent physical separation and parental practices which involve leaving a baby to 'cry out'. Parental behaviour should show low levels of sensitivity and responsiveness to infant signals.
2. The crying should reflect parental child care policies which differ from those of most parents. For instance, the parents may hold the view that responsiveness 'spoils' a baby. Parental or household variables which reduce responsiveness may also be common. For example, a high level of maternal depression or of family disorganisation may be found.

As with the temperament explanation of infant crying, the view that it is due to unresponsive parental care owes its origins to one path-finding study, Bell and Ainsworth's (1972) exploratory investigation of the effects of delayed parental response on crying levels in subsequent quarters of the first year. As with temperament research, too, the subsequent studies in this area have produced a more qualified and complex picture. The central weakness of Bell and Ainsworth's method was the confounding of maternal with infant variables: a mother cannot be responsive or unresponsive if an infant does not cry. Statistical methods are therefore needed which enable concurrent and consecutive relationships between maternal and infant behaviour to be separated out (Gewirtz and Boyd, 1977; Hubbard and van IJzendoorn, 1987, 1991). Although several research groups have reported findings at odds with Bell and Ainsworth's, Hubbard and van IJzendoorn's own (1991) study is by far the most conceptually and methodologically sound. Their finding was that delay in maternal response did *not* predict the duration of infant crying at subsequent ages. Maternal delay did predict the frequency of subsequent crying periods to a significant but limited degree (0.29). However, the relationship was the opposite of that reported by Bell and Ainsworth: delayed maternal response was associated with a *decreased* frequency of crying. An important finding was that delayed maternal response was common – mothers delayed response to 40 per cent of cry episodes – and was based on maternal interpretations of the reasons for the crying. Intense, painful-sounding crying was universally responded to immediately, while the mothers commonly adopted a wait-and-see strategy with more fretful behaviour. Hubbard and van IJzendoorn point out that such a 'differentiated response' – where parents take account of the intensity of a baby's crying and of contextual information about its probable basis – can be viewed in a positive light, since it affords the infant the opportunity to learn self-soothing strategies and to develop some independent control over its own environment.

As well as correcting the impression given by Bell and Ainsworth's (1972) research, Hubbard and van IJzendoorn's study draws attention to the difficulties involved in separating maternal from infant behaviour and in distinguishing inadequate from the normal range of 'good enough' parenting. As Hubbard and van IJzendoorn point out, it is the appropriateness of parental response which is the issue, rather than merely the promptness, and it is difficult to define appropriateness except in relation to an infant's needs. One way out of this apparent dilemma is to frame the question being asked in precise terms. On the one hand, it is not really in dispute that poor physical care will lead to raised levels of infant crying and it is at least plausible that neglectful psychological and social care will have a similar result. Indeed there is some evidence from socially 'at risk' samples that this is the case (Crockenberg and Smith, 1982; Anisfeld *et al.*, 1990). At the other extreme, there is little question that minor variations in how long a time parents take to respond to crying will lead to minor variations in infants' concurrent lengths of crying. There is again consistent evidence that this is the case (Bell and Ainsworth, 1972; Crockenberg and Smith, 1982; Hubbard and van IJzendoorn, 1991) and it is not surprising, given that infants often stop crying when responded to (Hubbard and van IJzendoorn, 1991). As Chapter 1 has indicated, neither of these phenomena, however, is really at issue. Rather, the question is whether parental care variations can account: (1) for the clustering of crying in the first three months, particularly in the evenings, in western infants generally; and (2) for the finding that a substantial minority of western infants cry for three or more hours per day, and remain relatively high criers for some months, in many cases in spite of the efforts of concerned parents in the normal community to resolve the crying.

Although none of the explanations for the evening crying peak considered in this chapter is satisfactory, it seems to be particularly difficult to account for it in terms of parental behaviour. To provide such an answer, it is necessary both to identify aspects of parental behaviour which are linked specifically to the evening and to show that they alter around the middle of the first year, when the evening crying peak diminishes. In contrast, studies of parental responsive care indicate either that this is stable over age, or that it changes gradually over the long term, partly in response to infant characteristics (Crockenberg and McCluskey, 1986; Hubbard and van IJzendoorn, 1991). Barr and Elias (1988) did find that the babies of La Leche League mothers who employed short interfeed intervals cried less during the daytime at two, but not at four, months than standard care infants. Barr *et al.* (1983) also found that breast-fed infants cried more frequently, but not for longer, in the first six weeks, while infants switched to formula feed at six weeks then cried less in the evening and more in the morning. Both these studies suggest that feeding interval or method may contribute to early crying and warrant further investigation. However, it is worth pointing out that moderated breast-feeding on demand (that is, with intervals longer than used by Barr and Elias's mothers) is a culturally based practice, rather than an indication of inadequate parental care. Since, too, this practice appears to be generally satisfactory, it is necessary to explain why some infants respond with crying to a practice to which other infants are able to adjust.

On the face of it, it is persistent crying which occurs repeatedly over the day, rather than crying at a particular time, which is more likely to result from inadequate care. As Chapter 1 indicates, this is also the pattern of crying most typical of infants referred for crying problems. Unfortunately, there is little direct evidence at present to show whether such parents employ distinct methods of care which might cause the crying. In principle, measures of the behaviour of parents who refer their babies for treatment of crying problems provide one possible source of such information, since a finding that referring parents behave abnormally at baseline, while treatments which normalise their behaviour result in diminished crying, would at least suggest a possible role for parental behaviour. Unfortunately, as Wolke (Chapter 3) points out, a striking feature of most studies which have sought to treat cases referred for early crying problems is the lack of any information about parental behaviour, either before or during the presumed period of intervention. The notable exception, Hunziker and Barr's (1986) study of supplementary carrying as an intervention, proved ineffective as a treatment where infants were already crying a great deal and also failed in a later study to reduce the level of crying in a general community sample. There is also a lack of evidence that relatively common maternal disturbances such as depression cause crying (Miller and Barr, 1991) and, in one study, maternal depression rates improved dramatically in response to reductions in crying (Pritchard, 1986).

Compared with this lack of direct evidence that parental behaviour is the initial cause of infant crying, there are several findings which weigh against this claim. One such finding, already noted, is that referring parents have often made extensive efforts to resolve their babies' crying (St. James-Roberts, 1992). A second is that firstborn babies do not cry more, so that parental inexperience – a powerful predictor of parental behaviour – is not a major factor in infant crying (Hubbard and van IJzendoorn, 1991; St. James-Roberts and Halil, 1991). A third is that there is a good deal of stereotyping in how women, at least, deal with infant crying, such that there seem to be more similarities than differences in the manoeuvres they use when confronted with a crying baby (Gustafson and Harris, 1990). Lastly, as noted earlier, both Bell and Ainsworth (1972) and Hubbard and van IJzendoorn (1987) have reported that mothers leave babies to cry for some time to see if they will settle on about 40 per cent of occasions, while such common variations in care seem to have little impact on the development of crying.

These findings against the view that parental behaviour is the cause of crying do not rule it out. Rather, the aim in this section has been both to highlight the complexity of the issues and evidence and to acknowledge that there is a contrary case. Where parents already have to contend with a baby who cries persistently and with the attendant feelings of distress and inadequacy, the implication that they are wholly or largely to blame for this state of affairs is unlikely to prove constructive. Given the authority which our society attaches to expert views, there is a need to avoid imputing blame to parents unless the evidence is unequivocal, and viable and effective remedies are available. Moreover, although research into the causal role of parenting behaviour needs to continue, there is also an argument that, particularly for immediate clinical purposes, this may not be the most salient focus. That is, rather than concentrating on the issue of what caused the crying in the first place, it may be more fruitful for therapeutic purposes to address the role of parental behaviour in responding to infant crying: that is, in maintaining or remedying it.

Implicit in this distinction between initial causes and the factors responsible for maintaining or developing crying is the belief outlined in the previous section of this chapter that crying needs to be approached as a developmental phenomenon. In addition, it is assumed that infants who cry persistently have special needs for environmental support, beyond those of most infants. This focus on infant 'special needs' has the advantage of avoiding blame, while directing attention towards the question of what positive action parents can take to meet their infant's needs. A further reason for this approach is that, compared with the evidence on parental care as the initial cause of crying, there is ample and consistent evidence of a role for parental behaviour in maintaining and developing it. In naturalistic studies, both Crockenberg and McCluskey (1986) and Engfer (1986) have found that infant irritability, maternal unresponsive attitudes and lack of social support interact in influencing the development of mother–infant interactions. Likewise, Maccoby *et al.* (1984) found that some mothers reduced their responsiveness to irritable twelve-month infants, while sons of mothers who exerted extra effort become less difficult at eighteen months, a finding which Fish *et al.* (1991) have more recently extended to infants in the first five months. Intervention studies, such as van den Boom's (1988) and Wolke *et al.*'s (1992), show, too, that when parents increase their responsiveness to infant crying, improved outcomes result.

Although a 'special needs' approach to infant crying is not likely to prove sufficient in the long term – since the initial causes of persistent crying need to be understood – it is a particularly attractive perspective for immediate, therapeutic purposes. As Wolke's chapter in this book illustrates, interventions which target parental behaviour provide a viable and cost-effective means of promoting infant adjustment irrespective of who or what initially caused the crying. Moreover, the view that an infant has special needs, and that parents can do something to help, can encourage parents to persist in their efforts instead of feeling helpless and demoralised.

Summary

The introduction to this chapter noted that crying is the final common pathway for a variety of infant needs and disturbances, so that a single explanation for persistent crying is unlikely to be found. It is clear that the research in this area is still some way from being able to say which factor, or interaction among factors, is responsible for persistent crying in any one case. None the less, a number of unifying themes which bear upon research and practice are discernible in recent studies.

1. Several of the explanations examined here propose that physiological reorganisations or disorders are at the heart of persistent crying, particularly during the first three months. Normal maturational processes are probably an important part of this picture, but are insufficient to account for it in isolation. There is evidence that gastrointestinal and autonomic nervous system disorders are involved in a minority of cases. It may well be that maturational

processes uncover and interact with the physiological vulnerabilities of individual infants to give rise to crying.

2. A developmental framework is helpful in drawing attention to the changes in the function of crying which occur as the infant develops from a reflexive to a social organism, capable of more complex emotions and of learning about the consequence of his/her actions. It follows that the causes of persistent crying will also change with age. Although there is little reason to believe that parental behaviour is a major initial cause of persistent crying, there is evidence that parents play a part in maintaining crying at older ages and that temperamental contributions to irritability increase as infants develop.

3. In conjunction with this developmental framework, a 'special needs' focus may be especially helpful for parents and for professional, therapeutic purposes. This focus involves concentrating not on the initial causes of crying, so much as on understanding the resources an infant currently needs in order to develop effective self-regulation. As well as removing the stigma of parental blame, this approach has the advantage of allying parents and professionals in planning positive steps which can be taken to meet the infant's developmental needs.

4. For research purposes, progress in disentangling causes will require more fine-grained measures, which distinguish between crying and irritability and which recognise the pattern and intensity of crying as important features. Bearing in mind the points made in Chapter 1, non-crying aspects of infant behaviour and parental and family variables will also need to be taken into account in explaining the social and clinical phenomenon of 'problem' infant crying.

References

Anisfeld, E., Casper, V., Nozyce, M. and Cunningham, N. (1990), 'Does infant carrying promote attachment? An experimental study of the effects of increased physical contact on the development of attachment', *Child Development*, 61, pp. 1617–27.

Barr, R.G. (1989), 'Recasting a clinical enigma: the case of infant crying problems (or colic)', in P.R. Zelazo and R.G. Barr (eds), *Challenges to Developmental Paradigms: Implications for theory, assessment and treatment* (Hillsdale, NJ: Lawrence Erlbaum).

Barr, R.G. (1990), 'The normal crying curve: what do we really know?', *Developmental Medicine and Child Neurology*, 32, pp. 356–62.

Barr, R.G. and Elias, M.F. (1988) 'Nursing interval and maternal responsivity: effect on early infant crying', *Pediatrics*, 81, pp. 529–36.

Barr, R.G., Kramer, M.S., Pless, I.B., Boisjoly, C. and Leduc, D. (1983), 'Feeding and temperament as determinants of early infant crying/fussing behavior', Presented in part at the Ambulatory Pediatric Association Meetings, Washington, DC, 5 May. Publications No. 00000, McGill University – Montreal Children's Hospital Research Institute.

Barr, R.G., McMullen, S.J., Spiess, H., Leduc, D.G., Yarenko, J., Barfield, R.,

Francoeur, T.E., and Hunziker, U.A. (1991a), 'Carrying as colic "therapy": a randomised controlled trial', *Pediatrics*, **87**, pp. 623–30.

Barr, R.G., Rotman, A., Yarenko, J., Leduc, D. and Francoeur, T.E. (1991b), 'The crying of infants with colic: a controlled empirical description', Presented at the combined meetings of the Ambulatory Pediatric Association and the Society for Pediatric Research, New Orleans, LA, 30 April –1 May.

Barr, R.G., Wooldridge, J. and Hanley, J. (1991c), 'Effects of formula change on intestinal hydrogen production and crying and fussing behavior', *Developmental and Behavioral Pediatrics*, **12**, pp. 248–53.

Bates, J.E. (1983), 'Issues in the assessment of difficult temperament', *Merrill-Palmer Quarterly*, **29**, pp. 89–98.

Bell, S.M. and Ainsworth, M.D.S. (1972), 'Infant crying and maternal responsiveness', *Child Development*, **43**, pp. 1171–90.

Bowlby, J. (1982), *Attachment and Loss, vol. 1: Attachment*, 2nd edn (New York: Basic Books).

Carey, W.B. (1984), '"Colic" – primary excesive crying as an infant–environment interaction', *Pediatric Clinics of North America*, **31**, pp. 993–1005.

Crockenberg, S.B. and McCluskey, K. (1986), 'Changes in maternal behavior during the baby's year of life', *Child Development*, **57**, pp. 746–53.

Crockenberg, S.B. and Smith, P. (1982), 'Antecedents of mother–infant interaction and infant irritability in the first three months of life', *Infant Behavior and Development*, **5**, pp. 105–19.

DeGangi, G., DiPietro, J.A., Greenspan, S.I. and Porges, S.W. (1991), 'Psychophysiological characteristics of the regulatory disordered infant', *Infant Behavior and Development*, **14**, pp. 37–50.

Emde, R.N., Gainsbauer, T.J. and Harmon, R.J. (1976), *Emotional Expression in Infancy: A biobehavioral study* (New York: International University Press).

Engfer, A. (1986), 'Antecedents of perceived behavior problems in infancy', in G.A. Kohnstamm (ed.) *Temperament Discussed* (Lisse: Swets-Zeitlinger B.V.).

Fish, M., Stifler, C.A. and Belsky, J. (1991), 'Conditions of continuity and discontinuity in infant negative emotionality: newborn to five months', *Child Development*, **62**, pp. 1525–37.

Fisichelli, V., Fisichelli, R., Karelitz, S. and Cooper, J. (1974), 'The course of induced crying activity in the first year of life', *Pediatric Research*, **8**, pp. 921–8.

Fox, N.A. (1989), 'Psychophysiological correlates of emotional reactivity during the first year of life', *Developmental Psychology*, **25**, pp. 364–72.

Gekoski, M.J., Rovee-Collier, C.K. and Carulli-Rabinowitz, V. (1983), 'A longitudinal analysis of inhibition of infant distress: the origins of social expectations?', *Infant Behavior and Development*, **6**, pp. 339–51.

Gewirtz, J.L. and Boyd, E.F. (1977), 'Does maternal responding imply reduced infant crying? A critique of the 1972 Bell and Ainsworth report', *Child Development*, **48**, pp. 1200–7.

Goldsmith, H.H., Buss, A.H., Plomin, R., Rothbart, M.K., Thomas, A., Chess, S., Hinde, R. and McCall, R. (1987), 'Roundtable: what is temperament? Four approaches', *Child Development*, **58**, pp. 505–29.

Gray, P. (1987), *Crying Baby: How to cope* (London: Wisebuy).

Gustafson, G.E. and Green, J.A. (1991), 'Developmental coordination of cry sounds with visual regard and gestures', *Infant Behavior and Development*, **14**, pp. 51–7.

Gustafson, G.E., and Harris, K.L. (1990), 'Women's responses to young infants' cries', *Developmental Psychology*, **26**, pp. 144–52.

Holmes, D.L., Reich, J.N. and Pasternak, J.F. (1984), *The Development of Infants Born at Risk* (Hillsdale, NJ: Lawrence Earlbaum).

Hubbard, F.O.A. and van IJzendoorn, M.H. (1987), 'Maternal unresponsiveness and infant crying: a critical replication of the Bell and Ainsworth study', in L.W.C. Tavecchio and M.H. van IJzendoorn (eds), *Attachment in Social Networks* (Amsterdam: Elsevier), pp. 339–75.

Hubbard, F.O.A. and van IJzendoorn, M.H. (1991), 'Maternal unresponsiveness and infant crying across the first 9 months: a naturalistic longitudinal study', *Infant Behavior and Development*, **14**, pp. 299–312.

Huntingdon, L., Hans, S.L. and Zeskind, P.S. (1990), 'The relation among cry characteristics, demographic varieties, and developmental text scores in infants prematurely exposed to methadone', *Infant Behavior and Development*, **13**, pp. 533–8.

Hunziker, U.A. and Barr, R.G. (1986), 'Increased carrying reduces infant crying: a randomized control trial', *Pediatrics*, **77**, pp. 641–8.

Hurry, J., Bowyer, J. and St. James-Robert, I. (1991), 'The development of infant crying and its relationship to sleep-waking organisation', *Society for Research in Child Development Abstracts*, **8**, p. 303.

Hyams, J.S., Geertsma, M.A., Etienne, N.L. and Treem, W.R. (1989), 'Colonic hydrogen production in infants with colic', *Journal of Pediatrics*, **115**, pp. 592–4.

Illingworth, R.S. (1985), 'Infantile colic revisited', *Archives of Disease in Childhood*, **60**, pp. 981–5.

Kagan, J. and Snidman, N. (1991), 'Infant predictors of inhibited and uninhibited profiles', *Psychological Science*, **2**, pp. 40–4.

Lamb, M.E. (1981), 'Developing trust and perceived effectance in infancy', in L.P. Lipsitt (ed.), *Advances in Infancy Research Vol. 1* (Norwood, NJ: Ablex).

Lester, B.M. (1985), 'There's more to crying than meets the ear', in B.M. Lester and C.F.Z. Boukydis (eds), *Infant Crying: Theoretical and research perspectives* (New York: Plenum), pp. 1–27.

Lester, B.M. and Boukydis, C.F.Z. (eds) (1985), *Infant Crying: Theoretical and research perspectives* (New York: Plenum).

Lester, B.M., Boukydis, C.F.Z., Garcia-Coll, C.T. and Hole, W.T. (1990), 'Colic for developmentalists', *Infant Mental Health Journal*, **11**, pp. 321–33.

Lester, B.M., Boukydis, C.F.Z., Garcia-Coll, C.T., Hole, W.T. and Peucker, M. (1992), 'Infantile colic: acoustic cry characteristics, maternal perception of cry, and temperament', *Infant Behavior and Development*, **15**, pp. 15–26.

Lothe, L., Ivarsson, S.A., Erman, R. and Lindberg, T. (1990), 'Motilin and infantile colic', *Acta Paediatrica Scandinavica*, **79**, pp. 410–16.

Lothe, L. and Lindberg, T. (1989), 'Cow's milk whey protein elicits symptoms of infantile colic in colicky formula-fed infants: a double blind crossover study', *Pediatrics*, **83**, pp. 262–6.

Maccoby, E.E., Snow, M.E. and Jacklin, C.N. (1984), 'Children's dispositions and mother–child interaction at 12 and 18 months: a short-term longitudinal study', *Developmental Psychology*, **20**, pp. 459–72.

Matheny, A.P. (1986), 'Stability and change in infant temperament: contributions from the infant, mother and family environment', in G.A. Kohnstamm (ed.) *Temperament Discussed* (Lisse: Swets-Zeitlinger B.V.), pp. 49–58.

Matheny, A.P., Riese, M.L. and Wilson, R.S. (1985), 'Rudiments of infant temperament: newborn to nine months', *Developmental Psychology*, 21, pp. 486–94.

Matheny, A.P., Wilson, R.S. and Nuss, S.M. (1984), 'Toddler temperament: stability across settings and over ages', *Child Development*, 55, pp. 1200–11.

Miller, A.R. and Barr, R.G. (1991), 'Maternal emotional state and infant behavior: are they related?', *American Journal of Disease in Childhood*, 145, pp. 4–21.

Parmelee, A.H. and Stern, E. (1972), 'Deveopment of states in infants', in C.O. Clemente, D.P. Purpura and F.E. Mayer (eds), *Sleep and the Maturing Nervous System* (New York: Academic).

Poole, S.R. (1991), 'The infant with acute, unexplained crying', *Pediatrics*, 88, pp. 450–5.

Prechtl, H.F.R. (1984), 'Continuity and change in early neural development', in H.F.R. Prechtl (ed.) *Continuity of Neural Functions from Prenatal to Postnatal Life* (Oxford: Black.vell), pp. 1–15.

Pritchard, P. (1986), 'An infant crying clinic', *Health Visitor*, 59, pp. 375–7.

Riese, M.L. (1987), 'Temperament stability between the neonatal period and twenty-four months', *Developmental Psychology*, 23, pp. 216–22.

Riese, M.L. (1990), 'Neonatal temperament in monozygotic and dizygotic twin pairs', *Child Development*, 91, pp. 1230–9.

St. James-Roberts, I. (1989), 'Persistent crying in infancy', *Journal of Child Psychology and Psychiatry*, 30, pp. 189–95.

St. James-Roberts, I. (1991), 'Persistent infant crying', *Archives of Disease in Childhood*, 66, pp. 653–5.

St. James-Roberts, I. (1992), 'Infant crying levels, and maternal patterns of care, in normal–community and clinically referred samples', in B.M. Lester, J. Newman and F. Pederson (eds), *Biological and Social Aspects of Infant Crying* (New York: Plenum), in press.

St. James-Roberts, I. and Halil, T. (1991), 'Infant crying patterns in the first year: normative and clinical findings', *Journal of Child Psychology and Psychiatry*, 32, pp. 951–68.

St. James-Roberts, I. and Wolke, D. (1988), 'Convergences and discrepancies among mothers' and professionals' assessments of difficult neonatal behaviour', *Journal of Child Psychology and Psychiatry*, 29, pp. 21–42.

St. James-Roberts, I. and Wolke, D. (1989), 'Do obstetric factors affect the mother's perception of her new-born's behaviour?', *British Journal of Developmental Psychology*, 7, pp. 141–58.

Thomas, A. and Chess, S. (1977), *Temperament and Development* (New York: Brunner/Maze).

Thomas, A. and Chess, S. (1986), 'The New York longitudinal study: from infancy to early adult life', in R. Plomin and J. Dunn (eds), *The Study of Temperament: Changes, continuities and challenges* (Hillsdale, NJ: Lawrence Erlbaum).

Thomas, A., Chess, S. and Birch, H.G. (1968), *Temperament and Behavior Disorders in Children* (New York: New York University Press).

Thomas, A., Chess, S. and Korn, S.J. (1982), 'The reality of difficult temperament', *Merrill-Palmer Quarterly*, 28, pp. 1–20.

Valman, H.B. (1989), 'Crying babies', in H.B. Valman (ed.), *The First Year of Life* (London: British Medical Association).

van den Boom, D. (1988), 'Neonatal irritability and the development of attachment:

observation and intervention', PhD Dissertation, University of Leiden, The Netherlands.

Wessel, M.A., Cobb, J.C., Jackson, E.B., Harris, G.S. and Detwiler, A.C. (1954),
'Paroxysmal fussing in infancy, sometimes called "colic"', *Pediatrics*, **14**, pp. 421–35.

Wolff, P.H. (1987), *The Development of Behavioral States and the Expression of Emotions in
Early Infancy: New proposals for investigation* (Chicago: University of Chicago Press).

Wolke, D., Gray, P. and Meyer, R. (1992), 'Helping parents to cope with their crying baby:
a controlled treatment trial', submitted.

Woodson, R.H., Blurton Jones, N.G., Da Costa Woodson, E., Pollock, S. and Evans, M.
(1979), 'Fetal mediators of the relationship between increased pregnancy and labour
blood pressure and newborn irritability', *Early Human Development*, **3**, pp. 127–39.

Worobey, J., and Lewis, M. (1989), 'Individual differences in the reactivity of young
infants', *Developmental Psychology*, **25**, pp. 663–7.

Zeskind, P.S. and Barr, R.G. (1992), 'Acoustic analysis of cries of infants with and without
colic', Presented to the Conference on Human Development, Atlanta, GA, April.

Zeskind, P.S. and Lester, B.H. (1978), 'Acoustic features and auditory perceptions of the
cries of newborns with prenatal and perinatal complications', *Child Development*, **49**,
pp. 580–9.

Chapter 3

The treatment of problem crying behaviour

Dieter Wolke, *University of Munich Children's Hospital*

Introduction

Crying is a young infant's first and most effective way of communicating needs to the caregiver. The infant's cry is a powerful signal, leading to physiological arousal, orienting and usually an urge to intervene in the adult caregiver (Brennan and Kirkland, 1983; Lounsbury and Bates, 1982; Wiesenfeld *et al.*, 1981; Boukydis and Burgess, 1982). These interventions can be manifold but feeding and carrying the infant are frequently chosen options (Ames *et al.*, 1984; Barr *et al.*, 1989; Bernal, 1972; Wright, 1989; Pridham *et al.*, 1989). Crying is adaptive in securing satisfaction of basic needs including hunger and closeness to the caregiver. Indeed, recent reseach has shown that babies which are placid and who rarely cry to indicate their need for food are at increased risk of poor growth, as parents are more frequently unaware of the need to feed at short intervals (Skuse *et al.*, 1991; Carey, 1985; DeVries, 1984).

In contrast, excessive crying is of great concern for parents who often feel desperate and find it difficult to cope with their infant (McKenzie, 1991; Farran and Farran, 1981; Gill, 1987; Wolke and Gray, 1989). In families with other psychosocial stressors, prolonged or unpleasant crying is often a factor precipitating physical abuse (Frodi and Lamb, 1980; Frodi, 1985; Kirkland, 1979). Excessive crying is one of the most frequent complaints of parents seeking help from paediatricians or other primary health professionals (Forsyth *et al.*, 1985a; Rubin and Prendergast, 1984). The need for help is often not matched, in the parents' opinion, by the advice given to them by health professionals (Wolke and Gray, 1989). As excessive crying is not associated with a known mortality or obvious morbidity, it is a condition traditionally thought of as transitory or self-limiting. However, as reviewed in

Chapter 1, there is now evidence that problems of several months' duration are quite common, with a minority of infants having long-term disturbance (see also van den Boom, 1988; Forsyth and Canny, 1991).

It is thus with some concern that, as in the field of sleep and feeding problems (Bax, 1989; Stores, 1990; Wolke, 1992), there are numerous papers communicating beliefs and wisdom on treatment approaches, but only few scientific and well-controlled evaluations of different treatments of excessive infant crying.

Definition of problem crying behaviour

Before reviewing the different treatment approaches, brief consideration should be given to the question of what is meant by problem crying behaviour (Wolke, 1988) in early infancy. That is, which factors in the infant's crying behaviour or pattern lead to the perception of a crying problem?

As Chapter 1 and other reviews (Wolke, 1990; Wolke and St. James-Roberts, 1986, 1987) have shown, maternal perceptions and interpretations of the intensity and amount of crying, as well as the maternal antenatal mental state (Zuckerman *et al.*, 1990, Parker and Barrett, 1992), are important factors determining maternal reports of crying behaviour. However, only in a minority of cases do mothers' false perceptions alone (i.e. seeking help in dealing with an infant who objectively cries little) lead to seeking help from professionals. St. James-Roberts and Halil (1991) and Wolke *et al.* (1993a) found in two independent large-scale studies that most mothers seeking help had infants who cried distinctly more than the 'average' infant. This has been further confirmed by St. James-Roberts *et al.* (1992a) who assessed infant crying by the use of voice-activated recordings of infants' cry vocalisations. They found that referred infants cried much more than non-referred community infants. In clinical practice it may thus suffice to consider any family as suffering from excessive infant crying if the parents perceive it as a problem (Schmitt, 1985). For clinical research purposes, however, there is mounting evidence that duration measures of crying should be the major defining feature of colic or crying problems in early infancy (Barr *et al.*, 1992), with Wessel *et al.*'s (1954) definition of colic as 'paroxysms of irritability, fussing, or crying lasting for a total of more than three hours a day and occurring on more than three days in any one week and that the paroxysms continue to occur for more than three weeks' most frequently referred to.

In summary, crying problems pertain mainly to excessive amounts of crying in the young infant. The crying has to exceed the parents' tolerance for this behaviour and produce prolonged stress before being considered (by the parents) as a crying problem.

A review of treatment approaches

Four different major approaches to the treatment of crying problems, described in the literature, can be distinguished:

1. Drug treatment.
2. Increased vestibular or vocal stimulation.
3. Dietary treatment.
4. Changes in parent–infant interaction.

In the following, mainly intervention strategies which have received some empirical evaluation of their effectiveness in reducing problem crying will be considered. The focus will be on crying problems in the young infant, i.e. the first six months of age (see Messer and Richards (Chapter 8) for a review of waking/crying problems in older infants).

Drug treatments

In the 1960s and 1970s, pharmacological agents were frequently prescribed to treat colic, in an attempt to alleviate the apparent pain in the infant and the tension in the family. Drugs with antispasmodic activity have been used most commonly, based on the assumption that colic is caused by spasms of the intestinal smooth muscles (Weissbluth *et al.*, 1984; Rubin and Prendergast, 1984). Four randomised controlled trials have been reported on the use of dicyclomine hydrochloride (DH) for the treatment of excessive evening crying (colic) (Illingworth, 1959; Grunseit, 1977; Weissbluth *et al.*, 1984; Hwang and Danielsson, 1985). The first two trials (Illingworth, 1959; Grunseit, 1977) claimed that DH was effective in the treatment of colic. However, as pointed out by Weissbluth *et al.* (1984), both studies used vague diagnostic criteria and neither showed a statistically significant reduction in infant crying. Weissbluth *et al.* (1984) designed a prospective randomised, double blind, placebo-controlled clinical trial using Wessel *et al.*'s (1954) definition of colic as the criterion for inclusion of infants into the trial (see above). Furthermore, crying amounts were systematically evaluated by using parents recording in standard diaries over a fourteen-day period. The findings were similar to the two previously reported, but less well evaluated, trials of crying. While 65 per cent of infants who had DH improved, only 32 per cent of those with placebo did (excluding those infants who did not complete the trial). The improvements in colic had no effect on either parent temperament ratings or parent reports of sleeping behaviour at four months of age.

Hwang and Danielsson (1985) queried the blindness of the previous trials as the placebos given did not closely resemble the taste of DH (as parents often taste their children's drugs). In a carefully controlled double blind cross-over trial with 30 infants they found that 25/30 infants improved with DH while 17 did with the placebo, a significant difference. 24-hour diaries further showed a significant reduction in crying with DH only, although the infants still cried much more (3.3 in 24 hours) post treatment than non-colicky infants of the same age (1.2 in 24 hours).

A further drug, dimethylpolysiloxsane (simethicone), which acts by changing the surface tension of mucus-entrapped gas bubbles allowing them to disperse, has frequently been used in Sweden to treat the assumed great deal of intestinal gas in colicky infants. Danielsson and Hwang (1985), in a double blind cross-over trial, evaluated the effectiveness of simethicone with 27 colicky infants. They found no differences between simethicone and placebo treament in observations, 24-hour diary or interview measures. Sixty-seven per cent of the parents reported that their infants improved during the placebo treatment period. Danielsson and Hwang (1985) concluded that the study provides no evidence that abdominal cramps caused by intestinal gas are a pathogenic mechanism. Rather, the high rate of improvement could be ascribed to a placebo (expectation) effect.

DH has been shown to be an effective symptomatic treatment (i.e. reducing evening crying) while the drug is given. It reduces crying but does not abolish it with crying levels, where measured systematically, remaining sustantially above community levels (Hwang and Danielsson, 1985). Side effects such as excessive drowsiness and associations with some cases of sudden infant death were queried (Illingworth, 1985), and the drug was withdrawn from the market in the mid 1980s. While DH is no longer recommended as a treatment for colic, it is also questionable whether antispasmodic and sedative treatment should be an option for intervention in colic, as evidence is lacking that excessive crying in infancy is the result of intestinal hypermotility. The therapeutic efficiency of DH may, in part, be explained by central effects (Hwang and Danielsson, 1985; Miller and Barr, 1991). It is noteworthy that a large number of infants improved also in the placebo condition, suggesting that psychological factors (i.e. changes in parental expectations) are an important ingredient in the pharmacological treatment of colic.

Increased vestibular or vocal stimulation

When evaluating the use of pacifiers, rocking, swaddling, increased carrying (vestibular stimulation) or vocal stimulation, a distinction has to be drawn as to whether these techniques are used to prevent crying, to reduce distress during specific painful medical interventions or for the treatment of infants with a crying problem.

Preventative strategies for 'normal infants'

Rocking. Rocking is the most widely studied strategy to reduce crying and has been used since the dawn of time. Experimental studies have usually been short term and have shown that rocking soothes babies immediately following the rocking. Studies of vestibular stimulation using rocking in the 1970s mainly employed mechanical rocking devices such as rockerboxes which could be oscillated at different speeds (frequency of rocking) (e.g. van den Daele, 1970; Ter Vrught and Pederson, 1973; Pederson, 1975; Pederson and Ter Vrught, 1973, DeLucia, 1969). The soothing effect of rocking appears to be augmented with increased frequency or rate (e.g. van den Daele, 1970; Ter Vrught and Pederson, 1973; Elliott *et al.*, 1988) and this effect is maximised when frequency and amplitude of rocking are both increased (Pederson and Ter Vrught, 1973). Byrne and Horowitz (1981) investigated specific rocking techniques (i.e. continuous versus intermittent), and moving of the infant in different directions (horizontally versus vertically) in regard to their effectiveness in soothing the infant. Generally, they found any rocking technique to soothe infants more rapidly than either just holding the infant upright on the shoulder (body contact) or leaving him to self-soothe. Intermittent forms of rocking lead post-intervention more frequently to bright-alert behaviour, and continuous rocking (in particular in the horizontal direction) to infant drowsiness. Rocking using oscillating waterbeds has also been frequently evaluated as a soothing technique for preterm infants in incubators (see Wolke, 1991a,b; Korner *et al.*, 1983; Barnard and Bee, 1983).

Carrying. Carrying, like rocking, is a common practice in many non-industrialised societies without alternative means of transport (Schieffenhövel, 1990). Baby carriers are commercially available and used regularly by a minority of mothers in western societies.

Hunziker and Barr (1986) evaluated the effect of increased infant carrying on the development of crying behaviour between three and twelve weeks in a randomised controlled trial. The intervention group mothers were asked to carry their infant at least three hours per day, independent of whether the infant was awake, crying or asleep. The control infants received only a child face stimulus placed in their cot. The crying behaviour in the intervention group was generally modified (Hunziker, 1990): (a) the daily amount of crying reduced; (b) the normal increase of crying from birth until six weeks of age (see Brazelton, 1962; Barr, 1990; Schölmerich and Hwang, 1991) was prevented; (c) evening crying was reduced; and (d) sleep behaviour was not influenced. The authors interpreted the effect of carrying to be due to a number of factors including rhythmic repetitive movements (rocking) and increased auditory stimulation or visual distraction, to name but a few. It may also have increased the sensitivity and immediacy of the mothers' response to their infant. The issue of what, precisely, was responsible for the improvements in infant crying is important, since two further attempts to use carrying to reduce crying have been unsuccessful. In a general community sample, St. James-Roberts *et al.* (1992b) were able to raise the amount mothers carried their babies to the same level as Hunziker and Barr (1986), but this did not lead to reduced crying. Barr *et al.* (1991) also used carrying as a treatment for problem crying (see below) and in this case too it failed to lower the infants' crying levels.

Swaddling and pacifier. Swaddling is an ancient practice and has been used in most cultures at one time or the other. Lipton *et al.* (1965) and Chisholm (1978) reviewed ethological and experimental observations of swaddling techniques for soothing infants. They concluded that swaddling, if initiated shortly after birth, may be effective in inducing sleep due to reduced motor activity. A recent controlled study compared swaddling with the use of a pacifier in two-week-old infants who underwent heel pricks and in two-month-old infants who received injections (Campos, 1989). The results indicated that the pacifier was more successful in terminating crying and reducing physiological distress than swaddling. While non-nutritive sucking has been described in studies with preterm infants (see Wolke, 1991a; Field *et al.*, 1982), controlled investigations regarding crying behaviour in normal infants are rare. However, Levine and Bell (1950), in an uncontrolled study, showed that increased pacifier use reduced excessive crying in most of 28 infants without adverse long-term effects such as thumbsucking. The study, however, used no standard measures of crying nor a control group.

Auditory stimulation. Auditory stimulation, in the form of so-called 'baby-soothing tapes' or white-noise baby soothers, is commercially available to the public. The first of the commercially available tapes included recordings of sounds resembling those found *in utero*.

Salk (1962) had suggested that the repetitive sound of the mother's heartbeat may be imprinted onto the foetus which later leads to soothing of the infant when exposed to it extra-uterine. DeCaspar and Fifer (1980) and DeCaspar and Sigafoos (1983) did indeed demonstrate that newborns show preference for the intra-uterine heartbeat of their mothers. However, it appears that any sound will calm babies more than no sound. Heartbeat similar to the mother's is no more effective than heartbeat dissimilar to that of the infant's mother for soothing (Smith and Steinschneider, 1975). There is some evidence that standard records of intra-uterine sounds calm babies. Murooka *et al.* (1975) showed that four out of five babies fell asleep when listening to intra-uterine sound records although the effectiveness of such noise has often been judged solely by mothers' reports (Callis, 1984). More systematic physiological studies have confirmed that exposure to continuous white noise led four-day-old neonates to reach quiet sleep sooner and that sleep duration was prolonged by 20 per cent (Murray and Campbell, 1971). A recent controlled study further showed that newborns on a postnatal ward fell asleep more frequently when listening to white noise (80 per cent of newborns) than if not exposed to white noise (25 per cent of control infants) (Spencer *et al.*, 1990). The study also indicated that white noise was only effective if the newborns were not hungry. Spencer *et al.* (1990) speculated that 'white noise probably acts by masking other external stimuli thereby removing such arousal stimuli and calming the baby' (p. 136). This masking effect may also explain mothers' reports that their infants calm when exposed to loud noises such as a vacuum cleaner, hair dryer or a washing machine (Paradise, 1966; Wolke and Gray, 1989, Spencer *et al.*, 1990). Any continuous, rhythmic noise seems effective in soothing newborn infants with white noise having being evaluated most thoroughly (Birns *et al.*, 1965; Brackbill, 1973).

Finally, a rather unusual approach to soothing infants was reported by Birns *et al.* (1966). They compared exposure to a 250 cps continuous tone, gentle rocking, a sweetened pacifier and immersing the infant's foot in water at 108 degrees Fahrenheit for their effectiveness in soothing young infants. They found that immersing the foot in warm water was most successful. This method is, however, not a very practical everyday approach to soothing.

In summary, a number of techniques soothe normal infants with vestibular stimulation having been tested most thoroughly. Furthermore, pacification effects appear to be cumulative: soothing is enhanced by stimulation of multiple sensory channels (Brackbill, 1971).

Treatment of problem criers
Most basic research on different soothing techniques has been conducted on normal, unproblematic infants. Frequently, the conclusion has been drawn that methods which work for infants with normal amounts of crying will also work for infants who cry excessively.

In an experimental study, Elliott *et al.* (1988), showed, indeed, that placing either normal criers or excessive criers in a motorised baby carriage for four minutes (40 or 57 rocks per minute) soothed both groups of infants equally well. The generalisation of this finding to the home setting is, however, misguided as illustrated by the study of Barr *et al.* (1991) who, encouraged by the findings in normal infants (Hunziker and Barr, 1986), conducted another randomised controlled trial. Subjects were 47 infants with colic (5–32 days of age). The trial compared standard advice (be responsive to crying, check nappy, pacifier, etc.) with a standard advice plus supplemental carrying group. No differences were found in the amount of crying during and after the intervention. In fact, at twelve weeks, standard advice infants cried significantly less than infants who received supplemental carrying (1.2 versus 1.9 hours per day). This finding shows that methods which are successful in general populations or in brief experimental settings are not necessarily appropriate and beneficial interventions for clinical populations. Barr *et al.* (1991) concluded that this apparent resistance to increased carrying (in marked contrast to normal infants) may be a defining feature of colic. However, the failure of carrying to be effective in preventing crying in other groups, mentioned earlier, needs to be borne in mind.

A third study, using a multiple baseline design across six infants, employed 'SleepTight', a device that vibrates the infant's crib to simulate the action of a car travelling at 55 mph (Sosland and Christophersen, 1991). Although crying amounts reduced in four of the six infants, the parents were not generally satisfied. Sosland and Christophersen (1991) concluded that 'SleepTight' may not be a viable means of managing infant colic.

Finally, Klougart *et al.* (1989) reported on a prospective, uncontrolled multi-centre chiropractor intervention study of 316 infants suffering from colic. The infants were between 2–16 weeks of age at the start of treatment, consisting of spinal manipulative therapy. Improvements were reported for 94 per cent of cases, whereby the average duration of colic reduced from 2.5 hours per day to 0.65 hours per day on day 14 according to maternal diary recordings. This finding is impressive at first sight but the lack of a control group and the highly selective group of mothers who consult chiropractors in private practice for crying problems allow no firm conclusions to be drawn. Furthermore, the so-called colic infants cried no more than normative data for this age group suggest is normal (Barr, 1990) and whether the chiropractors provided additional non-specific counselling is unknown.

Dietary treatment

Cow's milk allergy has recently been propagated as 'the' cause of colic. It is an explanation, popular both with certain researchers, parent magazines and parents. Finding an organic reason for excessive crying provides relief from any blame for parents. Recent work has indicated that parents use changes of formulas to deal with feeding or crying problems. Forsyth *et al.* (1985b) showed in a population study that 11 per cent of infants who had been breast-fed and 25 per cent who had been formula-fed since birth had been changed from cow milk formulas to so-called 'special formulas' (casein hydrolysate or soy protein formulas). Twenty-six per cent of mothers believed that their infants were allergic to cow's milk. Mothers who reported feeding or crying problems were most likely to change the formula (32 per cent). They believed significantly more frequently (than those who did not change the formula) that the problem was intrinsic to the infant and that the child had a disease or an illness.

Concern has been voiced regarding this trend. Taitz (1982) and Taitz and Wardley (1989) expressed the opinion that the overdiagnosis of cow milk hypersensitivity is a more serious threat than its underdiagnosis, in that it may have potential long-term effects on the child's rearing. If a child is thought to be allergic it may be falsely considered to be more vulnerable, or any subsequent behaviour may be falsely attributed to the allergy (Forsyth *et al.*, 1985b; Forsyth and Canny, 1991; Warner and Hathaway, 1984). Because of the concern voiced, dietary treatment will be considered here in detail.

There have been at least eight controlled studies and a number of field trials on the effect of the elimination of cow's milk protein as a treatment for colic or children's sleeping problems.

Dramatic reductions of colic have been reported in various studies by the research group from Malmö, Sweden (Lothe, Lindberg and Jakobsson). In field research, even 60 years ago, Shannon (1921) had suggested that allergic reactions to food antigens transmitted in maternal milk could cause colic. Jakobsson and Lindberg (1978) were the first to report on a scientific trial. Breast-feeding mothers who were 'informed that colic is a common symptom of allergy to cow's milk in infancy' (p.437) were asked to eliminate cow milk products from their diet. Twelve of the eighteen mothers had a family history of allergic disease. After one week of milk-free diet the infants were challenged again by introducing cow milk back into the mother's diet. A second challenge period followed. The article goes on to report on four patients whose colic disappeared during the cow-milk-free diet and where colic reappeared during challenges. In a second study, 65 infants fed cow's-milk-based adapted formulas took part in a 'double blind trial' (Lothe *et al.*, 1982). The infants were given a formula based on cow's milk for one week and a soy-based formula the next week. 'The mothers who fed their infants with small amounts of breast milk in addition to the formula were put on a diet free from cow's milk' (p. 8). Lothe *et al.* (1982) reported that seventeen infants (29 per cent) showed spontaneous recovery from colic, eleven infants improved when put on soy-based formula (18 per cent) and thirty-two infants (53 per cent) did not improve on either formula. However, when put on a casein-based formula (Nutramigen) all infants became symptomless within 48 hours.

These two studies were much quoted but the evidence is open to methodological criticism. To name just a few problems, both studies were non-blind (mothers were aware of the design and what kind of milk they administered; the challenges were also non-blind), non-randomised and had un- or poorly controlled trials. Furthermore, colic was defined clinically and by free parent reports (no systematic logs were used) (see Carey, 1989). All in all, the findings are equally well explained by parent expectations as they are by dietary effects.

Two recent studies by the Malmö group have addressed these earlier shortcomings with blind study designs. In the Jakobsson and Lindberg (1983) study, elimination of cow milk from the diet of breast-feeding mothers followed by its reintroduction, reportedly implicated cow milk as the cause of colic in twenty-three (35 per cent) of sixty-six colicky infants. Of the twenty-three mothers whose infants improved on the milk elimination diet, sixteen participated in a randomised, double blind cross-over trial and were given capsules containing whey protein or potato starch (placebo), followed by the free use of milk. Detailed perusal of the paper shows that six infants did not respond to either challenge, and five had no symptoms when milk was returned to the mothers' diet. Nine infants reacted only when their mother ingested whey capsules and with the open milk feeding (13.6 per cent of study group). Thus, using a blinded study approach, many fewer colicky infants were found to be allergic. Carey (1989) pointed to inconsistencies in the study report (number of infants in the challenges) and that nine infants cried more while seven cried less with cow's milk protein. Sampson (1989) further expressed doubt about the findings because of lack of information regarding crying times (the outcome measure colic was not defined objectively) and the suggestion that colic 'completely' resolved when the mothers were on a milk-free diet. Furthermore, there are doubts whether the samples were unselected. For example, in the first study (Jakobsson and Lindberg, 1978) the authors stated that twelve of the eighteen mothers had positive family histories of allergy (67 per cent), which does not represent the average colic population. It is likely that in the subsequent studies referral biases were present, in particular, that mothers of colic babies who had positive histories of allergy in their family sought help. Despite these biases, Jakobsson and Lindberg (1983) stated categorically 'We suggest a diet free of cow's milk for the mother as a first trial of treatment of infantile colic in breast-fed infants' (p. 270).

A fourth, most recent, study by Lothe and Lindberg (1989) tried to rectify much of the criticism directed against the previous studies. Twenty-seven patients with colic referred to the authors were first given cow's milk formula for a week (baseline) and then after a two-day wash-out period a cow's-milk-free diet (Nutramigen formula) for five days. On day 5, those infants who either got relief or were cured of the infantile colic (telephone interview) entered the double blind cross-over trial (twenty-four infants). The infants were challenged twice either with whey protein or a placebo (human albein powder) mixed into the Nutramigen. Eighteen of the twenty-four infants reacted to the challenge with increased crying, and symptoms such as gas formation and sleep problems were more common. This last study by the Malmö group used daily recordings of crying, but how this was done is not described in the paper, suggesting that general reports rather than diary logs were employed. Carey (1989) further remarked that in this latest study the definition of colic was changed from three hours per day crying to one and a half hours per day when it came to the cross-over trial. 'This shift meant that the diagnosis of colic could be expanded from 12 to 18 of those receiving whey protein capsules in their formulas' (p. 1125).

In stark contrast to these overwhelming reports of cow's milk allergy are the findings of studies which tried to replicate the results of the Malmö group. Double blind cross-over trials have been conducted by three independent groups in Finland (Stahlberg and Savilahti, 1986), New Zealand (Evans *et al.*, 1981) and the United States (Forsyth, 1989). Stahlberg and Savilahti (1986) and Evans *et al.* (1981) found no effect in eliminating and introducing cow milk back into the diet of colicky infants. However, some of the criticisms levelled at the Malmö group studies could also be addressed at these two studies, with doubts pertaining to the blindness in the Stahlberg and Savilahti (1986) study, in particular.

The study by Forsyth (1989) is the soundest study methodologically so far. He managed to circumvent most of the pitfalls encountered in studying infantile colic (Sampson, 1989). Seventeen colicky infants were alternatively fed Nutramigen or Nutragimen plus cow milk formula for four periods of four days each. Mothers recorded crying, fussing and colic in diaries for the sixteen-day study period. Significant decreases in crying and colic were seen with the initial formula change, and a significant decrease in colic and a possible decrease in crying were seen with the second change. However, no significant change in crying or colic was seen with the third formula change. Only two (11.8 per cent) of seventeen infants had clinically meaningful changes in crying with each formula change and could be considered as infants sensitised with adverse reactions to cow's milk.

Mixed evidence regarding the beneficial effect of a cow-milk-free diet, even in the offspring of families with positive histories of allergies comes from various field studies (Merrett *et al.*, 1988; Miskelly *et al.*, 1988; Bock, 1987; Iacono *et al.*, 1991) and a clinical trial (Taubman, 1988) which will be discussed later. The study by Merrett *et al.* (1988) investigated 487 babies who came from families with a positive history of allergies. Half of them were randomly assigned to a cow-milk-free diet and the other were fed with a soya substitute. No benefit resulted from withholding cow's milk, indeed symptoms were usually associated with this group. Similarly, in a study by Bock (1987), only a small group of children (8 per cent) were found to show reproducable reactions to various food stuffs.

In contrast, in another field trial in Belgium (Vandenplas *et al.*, 1988), a higher incidence of atopic manifestations (not necessarily crying) were found in infants whose family history was positive for atopic manifestations who received cow's-milk-based formula (18/45) versus infants on hypoallergenic formula formulations. The authors are cautious in interpreting their findings by stating that 'data on a larger population and double-blind investigations are needed before firm conclusions can be drawn' (p. 274). Similarly, a recent study from Italy found a high incidence of cow milk protein intolerance (CMPI) in formula-fed colicky infants confirmed by two successive challenges (71.4 per cent) (Iacono *et al.*, 1991). The study further indicated that nearly 20 per cent of CMPI infants had a positive anamnesis for atopy. The authors concluded that 'dietetic treatment should be the first therapeutic approach' (p. 332). The many methodological problems with this study, including a highly selected unrepresentative sample (70 infants from 240 infants diagnosed as suffering from colic in a gastroenterology outpatient clinic were non-randomly selected) and non-blind challenges with a clearly different-tasting formula containing soya, do not warrant the authors' over-enthusiastic conclusions.

It appears that more infants seem to suffer milk intolerance allergy when the study populations are recruited in specialist gastroenterology clinics (e.g. Jakobsson and Lindberg, 1983; Iacono *et al.*, 1991) than from general paediatric practitioner populations (e.g. Forsyth, 1989; Taubman, 1988). This suggests that sample preselection is a crucial factor for the interpretation of the findings.

The public discussion of cow milk allergy, the often unsubstantiated use of formula changes, based on controversial studies with many methodological shortcomings (see Sampson, 1989 or Carey, 1989) and the lack of evidence of serum markers for hypersensitivity to milk in colic babies (e.g. Liebman, 1981) urged the Committee on Nutrition of the American Academy of Pediatrics (1989) to state: '... there is no evidence to support the use of hydrolysate formulas for the treatment of colic, sleeplessness and irritability' (p. 1069). Taking into account the findings of the controlled and field trials, the current evidence suggests that food allergy may cause or be implicated in increased crying in a small subgroup of infants who cry excessively (10–15 per cent of such infants). If cow's milk intolerance has been established (multiple challenges), then parents should be informed that the cow's milk effect is likely to be short-lived and that the infant should be rechallenged at times (Bock, 1987; Forsyth, 1989) rather then being considered to suffer from a lifelong allergy (Hill and Milla, 1990).

Changes in parent–infant interaction

Many behavioural paediatricians and psychologists view persistent crying in the evening hours (colic) as due to the mismatch between the needs of a normal baby and the style of handling by the caregivers (e.g. Carey, 1984, 1989, 1990; Schmitt, 1986; Papousek, 1985; Pritchard, 1986; Hewson *et al.*, 1987). There are, however, divided opinions among the proponents of the parent-interaction hypothesis as to whether colic is caused, maintained or exacerbated by parental overstimulation, parent unintended reinforcement of crying behaviour or inadequate and insensitive responsiveness to the infant.

Reduction of overstimulation

Admitting older infants or toddlers into hospital if the parents are under extreme emotional strain has been proposed for infants with severe sleeping problems (Jackson and Rawlins, 1977; Bax, 1980). McKenzie (1991) observed that some babies referred to her and admitted to hospital, mainly because it was felt that a carer might harm the child, improved dramatically within a day or two. The effect of this dramatic treatment approach was attributed to the overstimulation the infants had received from their parents, who had worked (too) hard in trying to calm their infant. A study was initiated to investigate the overstimulation hypothesis. Mothers with infants with troublesome crying were asked to agree to randomisation to hospital admission versus home treatment. Randomisation was not successful as many parents refused hospital admission. However, thirteen of thirty-one mothers agreed hospital admission for an average of three days with only one mother being admitted with her infant. The other home treatment mothers were advised to reduce stimulation such as patting, frequent winding, jiggling the baby, etc. According to change ratings and cry time recordings, hospitalised infants cried much less than before admission (2.5 hours versus 12 hours). Those managed at home also improved significantly.

There are a number of problems with the study. Only half of the home-managed infant mothers returned complete diary records and had to be excluded from the study. Second, the initial reports of cry amounts were based on parent interviews and the post-treatment evaluations on diary records. Wolke *et al.* (1993a) and Klougart *et al.*'s (1989) findings indicate that parent reports may significantly overestimate cry times relative to systematic crying records.

In a second study, McKenzie (1991) evaluated how instructions to parents to reduce stimulation at home is helpful in eliminating excessive crying in comparison to a waiting (empathy) control group (parents who had an empathic interview and filled in a diary for a week and then received the same treatment) in a randomised trial. The changes in infant crying and mother's distress were evaluated using change ratings on eleven point rating scales. While both groups showed improvement, it was significantly higher in the advice group. Once the control mothers (after seven days) were also advised on reduction of stimulation, the infants improved further. Again, there are methodological problems with the second study. Most importantly, the outcome is based on parent ratings of change rather than more objective criteria of improvement such as diary measures. For example, Wolke and Gray (1989) found that parents report improvements in ratings which are not found in diary recordings of crying.

Lacking adequate evaluation, the findings are inconclusive. It is also not clear what mechanisms may explain the suggested effect of reduced stimulation. For example, is it the removal of reinforcers for crying in general (Larsson and Ayllon, 1990) or more sensitive (differential) responsiveness (Hubbard and van IJzendoorn, 1991) assisting the infant to find increased self-control in state regulation which may be operating in leading to the clinically observed reductions in crying? More stringent investigation documenting the actual changes in parenting behaviour is necessary to elucidate the mechanisms explaining the clinically observed effect of reduction of overstimulation (St. James-Roberts, 1992).

Differential reinforcement
Classical behavioural theory postulates that the frequency of inadequate behaviour (e.g. crying) is increased and the behaviour maintained by positive contingent reinforcement of this inadequate behaviour (Karoly, 1980). The behaviour is particularly resistant to change if the reinforcement is intermittent. To reduce operant crying, Etzel and Gewirtz (1967) proposed differential, that is, positive, reinforcement, with crying-incompatible behaviour such as smiling or eye contact being reinforced while crying is ignored (extinction). The success of this procedure has been described in case reports in older infants (e.g. temper tantrums, Williams, 1959). Etzel and Gewirtz also

described the success of this procedure in two case reports of a twenty-week-old and a six-week-old boy in the nursery setting. Furthermore, recent evidence from a longitudinal study of fifty mother–infant pairs showed that earlier maternal unresponsiveness (extinction) leads to less frequent crying later in the first half year of life but not necessarily to lower crying amounts (Hubbard and van IJzendoorn, 1991).

Taubman (1984) described the effect of an extinction procedure in six infants. The parents were instructed to put the baby in the crib upon crying for up to thirty minutes and to try to pick him up and calm him if he was still crying and, failing that, to return him to the crib until the infant fell asleep or three hours had passed. Taubman (1984) incorrectly labelled this procedure as a decreased stimulation condition (compare with McKenzie, 1991). No significant effects in reducing crying were found in this small group. As Larsson and Ayllon (1990) pointed out, this procedure maintained the infants' crying because, in classical operant behaviour theory terms, it scheduled intermittent reinforcement (parental attention) for persistent crying.

Larsson and Ayllon (1990) reported on a differential reinforcement schedule for the treatment of infantile colic evaluated by a multiple within subject reversal design. The major strategy consisted of (1) reinforcing the infants' adaptive behaviour with music plus parental attention and (2) inhibiting crying behaviour by following it with cessation of music plus brief time-out (placing the infant in a cot away from the parent). In addition, the relative effects of music in decreasing crying behaviour when music was (1) made non-contingent on behaviour and (2) when it was made contingent on quiet behaviour as a component of differential reinforcement were evaluated. The treatment of eight infants in three groups (3; 3; 2 infants) of 3–7 weeks of age diagnosed by a paediatrician as suffering colic was described. The effects of the treatments were evaluated using direct observation lasting one hour each on 1–4 days per week. The descriptive results indicate that contingent music combined with differential reinforcement increased adaptive and reduced maladaptive (crying) behaviour in infants. Although these case reports are impressive, no statistical evaluation is reported and is not possible due to the small group sizes. Second, it is not clear how much the infants cried per day, as the diagnosis was based on paediatricians' diagnosis alone and the observations lasted for only one hour per day.

Parent-sensitive responsiveness
Taubman (1984) evaluated the effectiveness of a parent counselling approach in his clinical practice. Twenty infants between one and eight weeks of age diagnosed clinically as suffering colic and eighteen control infants without colic problems participated in and completed the trial. Parents in both groups completed a 72-hour baseline diary which distinguished colic infants (Crying *M*: 2.6; SD: 1.1 hr/day) from control group infants (Crying *M*: 1.1; SD: 0.6 hr/day). The parents of the colicky infants were given instructions on how to

be more responsive to their infant's crying. These instructions were based on the premise that, in colicky babies, continuous crying may result when parents fail to respond to the baby's needs. In the treatment group only, the diaries were continued throughout the treatment period and reviewed frequently and new suggestions for the management of the infant were made, until a minimum of long episodes of crying was found on three consecutive days. These last three days of treatment served as outcome measures for the treatment group. The control group completed a second 72-hour diary two weeks after the baseline measure. The treatment infants improved significantly (post-treatment crying: M: 0.8; SD: 0.3 hr/day) and no differences from the control group were apparent anymore. The findings, although clinically impressive for the parental responses counselling approach, are open to methodological criticism. In particular, it is methodologically unsound to use improvement as the criterion to stop the trial and to use the three consecutive days showing reduced crying as post-treatment measures. This preprogrammes success if these measures are used as the outcome and it is unclear whether the reduction in crying was maintained once treatment stopped. Second, the design provides no evidence as to whether colicky infants not treated at all would have improved with time anyway. A non-treatment colicky infant group was missing. Finally, the amount of crying in the colicky group (2.6 hr/day) is hardly more than that found in naturalistic studies of crying behaviour of infants in the first three months in the United States and elsewhere (about 2 hours to 2 hours 30 minutes; Brazelton, 1962; Barr, 1990; Hunziker and Barr, 1986; St. James-Roberts and Halil, 1991) and less than that found in other clinical samples of colic infants (e.g. Weissbluth *et al.*, 1984; St. James-Roberts and Halil, 1991; McKenzie, 1991; Barr *et al.*, 1991; Wolke *et al.*, 1993a). The amount of crying in the control group was also much lower than that reported for the average crying of infants in the first eight weeks of life in naturalistic studies. It is thus questionable whether the trial pertains to a treatment study of excessive crying infants.

In a second clinical trial, Taubman (1988) compared two treatment approaches, parental counselling (group 1) versus elimination of cow's milk or soy milk protein from the diet (group 2) for colic. Twenty infants, less than eight weeks of age, with clinically diagnosed colic (crying of two or more hours per 24 hours) were randomly assigned to either of the two groups. After three days baseline diary assessment, group 1 received counselling and group 2 either received hydrolysed casein formula or nursing mothers were required to eliminate cow's milk from their diets. Both groups showed improvements against baseline over a nine-day period with the counselling group showing faster and greater change (group 1: 3.21 hr/day to 1.08 hr/day; group 2: 3.19 hr/day to 2.03 hr/day). In the second study phase, group 2 infants were re-exposed to cow's milk or soy protein and given counselling (like group 1 who finished the trial with phase 1). In this phase, counselling again decreased crying significantly from 2.09 hr/day to 1.19 hr/day. This better controlled study, rectifying many of the problems of the Taubman (1984) study, led Taubman (1988) to conclude 'that these data support the theory that for many infants with the infant colic syndrome the crying is a result of parental misinterpretation of infant cries and is not caused by milk protein allergy' (p. 756). Two remaining weaknesses are, first the lack of evidence that the parents implemented Taubman's instructions and that these were responsible for the changes in infant crying and, second, the omission of a control group which would have provided more conclusive information on whether untreated infants would have improved as much as group 2 infants over the nine-day period.

Wolke *et al.* (1993b) evaluated a developmental programme (P1) in a nationwide controlled-treatment trial with colic infants (2–6 month olds), described here, and a second cohort of 6–18 month olds, described elsewhere (Wolke and Gray, 1989), in Britain. P1 was compared to a second 'empathy-feeling sharing' treatment approach and a non-treatment control group (C) of excessive criers. The P1 programme is described in detail later in this chapter; in the P2 condition the counsellors shared their feelings with the mothers and talked about what had helped them in the past dealing with their own crying infant. All counselling took place on the telephone, was brief (usually three treatment contacts) and was carried out by trained lay counsellors of the parents self-help group CRYSIS. Infant crying was assessed with a 7-day diary at baseline (see below and Fig. 3.2) and 3.5 months later at follow-up. Only infants crying three or more hours per day, on average, over the 7-day baseline diary period, and where the problem had lasted for more than one month, entered the trial (P1: N:21; P2: N:27; C: N:44). There were no differences in the amount of crying or in sociodemographic indices between the groups at baseline. The results showed that infants in all three groups cried significantly less 3.5 months later. However, as Fig. 3.1 shows, crying reduced significantly more in the developmental behavioural treatment group infants P1 (baseline fuss/cry M:345.8 min;

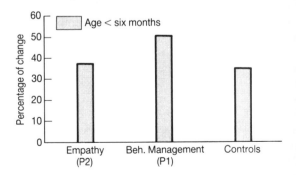

Figure 3.1 Reduction in cry behaviour from baseline (expressed as percentage of change) (Wolke *et al.*, 1993b).

post-treatment fuss/cry *M*: 169.4 min, improvement 51 per cent) than in the P2 condition (empathy-feeling sharing reduction, baseline fuss/cry *M*: 365.6 min, post-treatment fuss/cry *M*: 228.5 min, improvement 37.5 per cent) or control group (baseline fuss/cry *M*:343.0 min; post-treatment fuss/cry *M*: 222.11 min, improvement 35.2 per cent). Furthermore, mothers in both treatment groups (P1; P2) were asked whether the treatment had helped them in 'reducing the crying and sleeping problem', 'in improving the parent–child relationship' and 'coping with her infant'. Mothers reported significantly more improvements in the P1 than P2 condition. The mothers also evaluated the counsellors in P1 more positively although they were the same in P1 and P2.

Wolke *et al.*'s (1993b) study demonstrates that a brief developmental behavioural management counselling on the telephone is successful in reducing excessive crying in young infants and that this reduction is maintained over a three-month period. The mothers are pleased with the intervention, perceive improvements and are less anxious and depressed (see also Downey and Bidder, 1990). Being empathetic, sharing feelings and exchanging experiences, in contrast, has no greater effect than not treating the mothers at all. It is notable that many parents in the control group commented that completing the baseline diary and several questionnaires was helpful in understanding and dealing with the crying. This indicates that the baseline diary itself may have therapeutic qualities.

Finally, a treatment study, by van den Boom (1988), provides direct evidence of the interrelationship between the infant characteristic irritability (poor state control and crying to minimal stimuli), its effect on parent responsiveness to the child and adverse outcome. She tested whether a brief intervention consisting of three home visits between six and nine months of age would result in improved parent–infant interactions, reduced infant crying and more secure infant attachment. The investigation (not primarily a crying treatment study) addressed this older infant group as this age is considered as an important period for attachment formation. Van den Boom (1988) used an innovative four-group research design adapted with small changes from that proposed by Solomon and Lessac (1968) and illustrated in Table 3.1. The main aim of this design is to test whether the pretest observation itself already has an independent or interactive effect on the outcome. Second, including a control group (group III) which receives as many visits as the experimental groups but for observation only, allows for the fact that getting attention alone would already have a positive effect on maternal behaviour and subsequently infant behaviour. Altogether 100 infants, identified as highly irritable in the newborn period (from 588 infants tested) were assigned to one of the four groups (25 infants each). The experimental condition consisted of reinforcing the mother's sensitive responses to infant signals, to enhance her confidence and to discuss sensitive response strategies for problematic infant behaviours. The mother–infant

Table 3.1 The four-group design proposed by Solomon and Lessac (1968) employed by van den Boom (1988) in her intervention study.

	Pretest	Experimental treatment	Post-test
Experimental groups			
Group I	X	X	X
Group II		X	X
Control groups			
Group III	X	O	X
Group IV			X

dyads were evaluated shortly after termination of the intervention (nine months of age) and at twelve months of age by 'blind' observers. The results were clear cut in showing that programme mothers (groups I and II) were more responsive, more cognitively stimulating and more controlling of their infant's behaviour. The programme infants were more sociable, explored more and cried less than control infants. At twelve months of age, using the Ainsworth *et al.* (1971) strange situation, 14 of 50 control infants in contrast to 34/50 treatment infants were classified as securely attached. The major difference appeared to be that control mothers attended mainly and then angrily to negative (crying) infant signals, while treatment mothers learned to respond positively to both positive and negative infant signals. Pretest observations or observation visits *per se* (group III) showed no or only minimal effects on the outcome measures.

This study is both elegantly conceived and methodologically sound. Apart from demonstrating the effect of home visits on infant crying and mother–infant interaction, it indicates that infant characteristics such as irritability in combination with maternal characteristics (e.g. unresponsiveness) or maternal interpretations of this behaviour (Wolke and St. James-Roberts, 1986) lead to adverse outcome and poorer mother–child relationships.

Conclusions

In summary, the approaches which will be named provocatively as 'easy recipe' approaches (i.e. drug treatment, increased carrying, hospital admission) are either controversial in their findings (hospital admission), not reliable (increased carrying) or only successful while treatment lasts (e.g. drugs). Of the different treatment approaches there are currently two main contenders promising to be successful in reducing crying amounts in some or most young infants: changes in parent–infant interaction and cow's milk elimination.

The hypothesis that excessive crying in young infants is partly due to or maintained by problems in the signalling of a particular infant and the interpretations and interventions of his parents, has been supported by the reported recent studies. There is, however, some controversy about the exact mechanisms and intervention stategies in changing parent–infant interaction (e.g. classical behavioural versus increased sensitive responsiveness approach). Methodological problems have been highlighted in some of the parent counselling studies, indicating the need for better controlled clinical trials.

Despite the heated discussion regarding the milk allergy hypothesis it appears established that cow milk elimination is successful in a small minority of cases in the treatment of excessive crying. Cow milk elimination should *not* be the first treatment option because of its limited success in the majority of cases and the danger of building up the idea in the parents' minds that the infant is vulnerable or ill (Forsyth and Canny, 1991; Taitz and Wardley, 1989).

Overall, excessive crying in different infants is probably caused by several factors. Thus no single approach is likely to be successful in all cases. From the current evidence, an eclectic approach adapted to the individual family appears to be the most promising. It should thus not be disconcerting in clinical practice if parental counselling is combined with dietary management where changes in parent–infant interaction alone do not lead to improvement in crying and where atopic illnesses are prevalent in the family.

Future directions

There are a number of theoretical and methodological issues which are deficient in the currently published treatment work and which should be addressed in future work with crying babies.

1. Excessive crying is treated as being synonymous with colic, persistent crying paroxysms in the evening in infants in the first 3–5 months of age. This is a misleading assumption. Most work has acknowledged that those infants crying much in the evenings usually also cry more than 'non-colicky' babies at other times of the day (see Wolke and Gray, 1989; St. James-Roberts and Halil, 1991). The duration of crying should be the defining criterion for treatment studies and not paediatric diagnosis, abdominal distension or other such criteria *per se*. There is increasing evidence that Wessel *et al*.'s (1954) criterion may be a sensible distinction for excessive versus not excessive criers in early infancy (Barr *et al*., 1992) and should be adopted in clinical trials. Studies reporting on infants crying less than three hours on average may be considered preventive rather than treatment studies and should be interpreted cautiously when generalised to excessive cry populations.

2. It is often overlooked that crying problems are also a concern of parents in older infants and toddlers (e.g. temper tantrums, bedtime problems, night waking). Systematic studies on crying behaviour and treatment of crying problems in infants between four and eighteen months are generally lacking with few exceptions (van den Boom, 1988; Wolke and Gray, 1989). This is

most surprising, as crying problems in this age group are as, or even more, likely to be persistent and to predict later behaviour and sleeping problems (e.g. McDevitt, 1986; Snow *et al.*, 1980; Jenkins *et al.*, 1984).

3. While basic research on the normative development, the neuro–physiological basis of crying and the adult perception of crying has taken a developmental standpoint, this is lacking in most treatment approaches. Developmental principles have been acknowledged implicitly only in the parent–infant interaction approach and non–empirical psychoanalytical writings on excessive crying. A holistic view of crying, considering crying and its relationship to other domains of development of competence such as feeding, sleeping, cognitive and socioemotional development, is needed (see Wolke, 1992; van den Boom, 1988).

4. Where changes in parental behaviour are required (e.g. dietary changes in breast-feeding mothers; increased carrying, changed responsiveness, etc.), control via direct observation techniques would be desirable to ascertain whether changes in these target behaviours have really been implemented (St. James-Roberts, 1992). In particular, where negative results are reported, it is unclear whether these cannot be attributed to a lack of implementation of treatment suggestions rather than to treatment failure. It is hoped that improved methodologies of evaluation studies and improved training of primary healthcare workers will lead to more effective interventions, founded in developmental theory. The health practitioner can be certain of gratitude from stressed parents if he or she can assist in alleviating excessive infant crying.

Treatment in practice – an individualised developmental treatment approach

In the following, a treatment approach is outlined which has been empirically evaluated (described in the section 'Parent-sensitive responsiveness', pp. 62–3), and may be implemented by health visitors, general practitioners, community paediatricians or clinical psychologists. The approach is deduced from findings of previous treatment research and basic research on crying behaviour (see St. James-Roberts (Chapter 1); Wolke, 1986) and further based on research and clinical work in other domains, mainly the development of state control, sleeping and feeding patterns (see Skuse and Wolke, 1992; Wolke and Skuse, 1992; Wolke and Eldridge, 1992; Wolke, 1993a,b).

Premises

The basic premises of our approach are:[1]

1. The type, amount, frequency and biological and social meaning of

crying change with age; i.e. there is 'lawful' developmental change. Crying under the age of six months is mainly under biological control (Lester *et al.*, 1989). The infant is not crying to assert himself or to get at the parents but is going through a period of acquiring 'basic' behavioural organisation including diurnal and circadian wake and sleep periodicity acquisition, management of new feeding patterns, etc. (Wolke and Skuse, 1992; Wolke, 1993b; Wolff, 1987; Sander, 1987; Miller and Barr, 1991). Crying becomes a means of self-assertion after roughly the age of six months with the understanding of intentions (Trevathen, 1987; Lewis, 1992) and the discrimination of social responsiveness in the young infant between the primary caregiver and others not present. The older infant uses crying as a means of getting attention or to press for a certain social goal (e.g. temper tantrums, night crying, etc.). This is the time when bedtime problems and night waking re-occur in infants who slept through the night before (e.g. Moore and Ucko, 1957; Anders and Keener, 1985).

2. There is a developmental tendency for infants to modulate, tolerate and endure experiences of negative affect and to acquire other means than crying in communicating needs (Demos, 1986). Crying has both a practical component (i.e. communicating hunger) and an affective component, communicating about an inner state of what the infant is feeling. The parents' role is to recognise the communication, to support the internal control and to provide alternative means (other than crying) of expressing needs and affect.

3. Individual differences in the cry signals (acoustic qualities), amount and frequency of crying are apparent, particular in young infants (van den Boom, 1988; St. James-Roberts and Wolke, 1988; St. James-Roberts and Halil, 1991). These individual differences are embedded in differential rates of developmental change (i.e. maturational changes in state control) and only influenced by perinatal factors in the short term (St. James-Roberts and Wolke, 1989).

4. There are individual differences in caregiver perceptions of crying (e.g. tolerance for crying) and in the behavioural repertoire and flexibility in applying different strategies (Shaw, 1977; van den Boom, 1988; Crockenberg, 1981, 1986; Sander, 1969). For example, as documented by Wolke and St. James-Roberts (1986, 1987) and Wolke (1990), parents have styles of attributions for crying, greatly variable behaviour repertoires (e.g. some mothers just use feeding indiscriminately when the infant cries) and differ in their flexibility in changing strategies. Furthermore, mothers' depression influences their ability to deal with a crying infant (Cutrona and Troutman, 1986). Depression may occur as a result of the crying but, as Zuckerman *et al.* (1990) and Vaughn *et al.* (1987) have shown, depression and anxiety in pregnancy often precede crying problems or perceptions of infant difficulties in early infancy.

5. Environmental and social factors partly determine or maintain certain intervention strategies. For example, living in a small apartment in a block of

apartments puts much more pressure on the mother to keep her infant quiet than living in a detached house.

6. Crying problems are intensified or maintained by the parents due to inappropriate management and support for internal control of the infant according to his/her current developmental requirements.

The treatment process

These premises have important implications for treatment. It follows that it has to be developmentally oriented, individualised and to use a 'no-blame' principle; neither parent nor infant are blamed for the problem. The treatment of excessive persistent crying involves four steps.

The initial assessment

Step 1 Learning about the problem – the behaviour diary. Parents should complete a detailed behaviour diary including the following behaviours: crying, fussing (fretting), feeding and sleeping for 15 minute intervals for 24 hours for 7 days. Furthermore, a column should be provided for the parents to indicate the interventions they used when trying to console their infant. An example of such a diary is shown in Fig. 3.2.

The following information should be extracted from the diary:

1. How much does the infant actually fuss and cry?
2. Is there a pattern of crying and fussing (e.g. diurnal; situation specific, etc.)?
3. Are there particular strategies which work best in comforting the infant?; how many different strategies are used?; are there interventions which are overused (e.g. feeding)?
4. Is there a pattern of feeding and sleeping (i.e. is there a predictable daily routine with regular bedtimes, daytime naps, feeds, etc.)?
5. How much social stimulation does the infant receive?; is it too little (note sleep intervals and total sleep time) or too much (note indications of interventions)?

Step 2 The family situation
1. Build a picture of the psychological status of the mother, the partner relationship and social support available (e.g. using standardised measures; see Wolke *et al.* (1993b)). This partly determines which treatment suggestions are likely to be put into practice by the parents (Wolke, 1993b).
2. Explore whether parental, family or social support problems are a reaction to the child's crying behaviour (e.g. a crying baby can wear you out, affect the marriage and friendships) or were present before the arrival of the child.

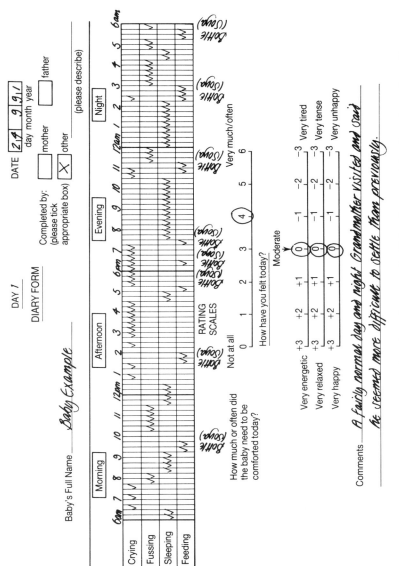

Figure 3.2 Example of a 24-hour diary for a three-month-old boy (name and date have been changed).

The information gathered in step 1 and 2 is used to build a picture of the infant's and parents' behaviour pattern. Hypotheses are formulated and probed in the first treatment session (after the initial assessment). All infants enrolling in the treatment programme should have a medical check-up to exclude possible medical problems contributing to the crying problem. It should always be probed how emotionally intense (anger, rising tension, etc.) the parents' reaction to the infant's crying is. The risk of possible physical abuse should be judged and appropriate precautions considered.

The actual intervention

Step 3 Planning some strategies
1. What to tackle first? Build a hierarchy of problems (there are often associated sleeping or feeding problems in persistent excessive cry infants). Tackle the problem that is most important to the parents. It should be a goal that can be reached realistically within a time period of less than three weeks.
2. Get a commitment from both parents and agreement for consistency in tackling the problem from both partners.
3. Discuss with the parents the consequences of reduced crying (e.g. secondary loss such as feeling less needed, loss in sympathy from partner or friend, etc.).

Useful treatment interventions

The young infant (< 6 months)[2]. The different strategies have one aim: find the best way of providing the young infant with external means in supporting the infant's internal behavioural organisation.

1. Provide information about normal crying patterns, i.e. young infants cry between 1.5–2.5 hours per 24 hours with 40 per cent crying most in the evening hours. This is often reassuring for parents with 'objectively' no or little crying problems.
2. Establish a daily routine and pattern of activities, for sleeping and feeding behaviour (this assists the building of internal control and enhances the predictability of caregiving actions for the infant).
3. Reduce overstimulation, or in the case where parents expect the infant to sleep more than developmentally adequate or necessary (i.e. under-stimulated), give advice on techniques for playful and moderately arousing interaction.
4. Discuss feeding techniques and the use of breast and bottle feeding as an (inadequate) soothing technique. Feeding should not be the 'unreflected' first option when the infant is crying. A repertoire of techniques for soothing infants should be discussed or demonstrated, suitable to the individual infant.

5. Explain to the parents that state control is the first acquisition of self-competence by the infant. Intervening at every fret of the infant never allows the infant to self-soothe. On the other hand, the parents should not leave the infant to cry it out. Waiting one to two minutes before intervening is advised, although this rule is dependent on the intensity and reason for the crying (see Demos (1986) and Hubbard and van Ijzendoorn (1991) for a discussion).
6. Occasionally, especially when the mother suffers severe depression or severe relationship problems, individual or partner counselling may be indicated.

Step 4 Treatment evaluation. Any treatment should not only be evaluated at the end of the treatment but also some months later to obtain feedback on whether the initiated changes have been maintained, using structured diaries or a short interview with the parents on subsequent clinic visits.

Notes

1. A Parent Self-Help Manual (Wolke and Gray, 1988) is available from the author.
2. The treatment of crying problems in older infants is described in the Parent Self-Help Manual by Wolke and Gray (1988) and in Wolke (1993b).

References

Ainsworth, M.D.S., Bell, S.M. and Stayton, D.J. (1971), 'Individual difference in strange situation behavior of one year olds', in H.R. Schaffer (ed.), *The Origins of Social Relations* (London: Academic).

Ames, E.W., Gavel, S., Khazie, S. and Farrell, T. (1984), 'Mothers' reports of infant crying and soothing', Paper presented at the 4th International Conference on Infant Studies, New York, April.

Anders, T.F. and Keener, M.A. (1985), 'Developmental course of nighttime sleep–wake patterns in full-term and premature infants during the first year of life', *Sleep*, 8, pp. 173–92.

Barnard, K.E. and Bee, H.L. (1983), 'The impact of temporally patterned stimulation on the development of preterm infants', *Child Development*, 54, pp. 1156–67.

Barr, R.G. (1990), 'The normal crying curve: what do we really know?', *Developmental Medicine and Child Neurology*, 32, pp. 356–62.

Barr, R.G., Kramer, M.S., Pless, I.B., Boisjoly, C. and Leduc, D. (1989), 'Feeding and temperament as determinants of early infant crying/fussing behavior', *Pediatrics*, 84, pp. 514–21.

Barr, R.G., McMullen, S.J., Spiess, H., Leduc, D.G., Yarenko, J., Barfield, R., Francoeur, E. and Hunziker, U.A. (1991), 'Carrying as colic "therapy": a randomized controlled trial', *Pediatrics*, 87, pp. 623–30.

Barr, R.G., Rotman, A., Yarenko, J., Leduc, D., and Francoeur, T.E. (1992), 'The crying of infants with colic: a controlled empirical description', *Pediatrics*, 90, pp. 14–21.

Bax, M.C.O. (1980), 'Sleep disturbance in the young child', *British Medical Journal*, **280**, pp. 1177–9.

Bax, M.C.O. (1989), 'Eating is important', editorial, *Developmental Medicine and Child Neurology*, **31**, 285–6.

Bernal, J. (1972), 'Crying during the first 10 days of life and maternal responses', *Developmental Medicine and Child Neurology*, **14**, pp. 362–72.

Birns, B., Blank, M. and Bridger, W.H. (1966), 'The effectiveness of various soothing techniques on human infants', *Psychosomatic Medicine*, **28**, pp. 316–22.

Birns, B., Blank, M., Bridger, W.H. and Escalona, S.K. (1965), 'Behavioral inhibition in neonates produced by auditory stimuli', *Child Development*, **36**, pp. 639–45.

Bock, S.A. (1987), 'Prospective appraisal of complaints of adverse reactions to foods in children during the first 3 years of life', *Pediatrics*, **79**, pp. 683–8.

Boukydis, C.F.Z. and Burgess, R.L. (1982), 'Adult physiological response to infant cries: effects of temperament of infant, parental status, and gender', *Child Development*, **53**, pp. 1291–8.

Brackbill, Y. (1971), 'Cumulative effects of continuous stimulation on arousal levels in infants', *Child Development*, **42**, pp. 17–26.

Brackbill, Y. (1973), 'Continuous stimulation and arousal level in infancy: effect of stimulus intensity and stress', *Child Development*, **46**, pp. 43–6.

Brazelton, T.B. (1962), 'Crying in infancy', *Pediatrics*, **29**, pp. 579–88.

Brennan, M. and Kirkland, J. (1983), 'Perceptual dimensions of infant cry signals: a semantic differential analysis', *Perceptual and Motor Skills*, **57**, pp. 575–81.

Byrne, J.M. and Horowitz, F.D. (1981), 'Rocking as a soothing intervention: the influence of direction and type of movement', *Infant Behavior and Development*, **4**, pp. 207–18.

Callis, P.M. (1984), 'The testing and comparison of the intra-uterine sound against other methods for calming babies', *Midwives Chronicle*, **97**, pp. 336–8.

Campos, R.G. (1989), 'Soothing pain-elicited distress in infants with swaddling and pacifiers', *Child Development*, **60**, pp. 781–92.

Carey, W.B. (1984), '"Colic" – primary excessive crying as an infant–environment interaction', *Pediatric Clinics of North America*, **31**, pp. 993–1005.

Carey, W.B. (1985), 'Temperament and increased weight gain', *Developmental and Behavioral Pediatrics*, **6**, pp. 128–31.

Carey, W.B. (1989), 'Cow's milk formula and infantile colic', letter, *Pediatrics*, **84**, pp. 1124–5.

Carey, W.B. (1990), 'Infantile colic: a pediatric practitioner-researcher's point of view', *Infant Mental Health Journal*, **11**, pp. 334–9.

Chisholm, J.S. (1978), 'Swaddling, craddleboards and the development of children', *Early Human Development*, **2/3**, pp. 255–75.

Crockenberg, S.B. (1981), 'Infant irritability, mother responsiveness, and social support influences on the security of infant–mother attachment', *Child Development*, **52**, pp. 857–65.

Crockenberg, S.B. (1986), 'Are temperamental differences in babies associated with predictable differences in caregiving?', in J.V. Lerner and R.M. Lerner (eds), *Temperament and Social Interaction in Infants and Children*, New Directions for Child Development No. 31 (San Francisco: Jossey-Bass), pp. 53–73.

Cutrona, C.E. and Troutman, B.R. (1986), 'Social support, infant temperament, and parenting self-efficacy: a mediational model of postpartum depression', *Child Development*, **57**, pp. 1507–18.

Danielsson, B. and Hwang, C.P. (1985), 'Treatment of infantile colic with surface active substance (simethicone)', *Acta Paediatrica Scandinavica*, 74, pp. 446–50.

DeCaspar, A.J. and Fifer, W.P. (1980), 'Of human bonding: newborns prefer their mothers' voices', *Science*, 208, pp. 1174–6.

DeCaspar, A.J. and Sigafoos, A. (1983), 'The intrauterine heartbeat: a potent reinforcer for newborns', *Infant Behavior and Development*, 6, pp. 19–25.

DeLucia, L. (1969), 'The influence of rocking stimulation on the crying behavior of infants', *Bulletin of Brown University Child Study Center*, 3, pp. 1–2.

Demos, V. (1986), 'Crying in early infancy: an illustration of the motivational function of affect', in T.B. Brazelton and M.W. Yogman (eds), *Affective Development in Infancy* (Norwood, NJ: Ablex Publishing Corporation).

DeVries, M.W. (1984), 'Temperament and infant mortality among the Masai of East Africa', *American Journal of Psychiatry*, 141, pp. 1189–94.

Downey, J. and Bidder, R.T. (1990), 'Perinatal information on infant crying', *Child: Care, Health and Development*, 16, pp. 113–22.

Elliott, M.R., Fisher, K. and Ames, E.W. (1988), 'The effects of rocking on the state and respiration of normal and excessive criers', *Canadian Journal of Psychology*, 42, pp. 163–72.

Etzel, B.C. and Gewirtz, J.L. (1967), 'Experimental modification of caretaker-maintained high-rate operant crying in a 6- and 20-week-old infant (Infans tyrannotearus): extinction of crying with reinforcement of eye contact and smiling', *Journal of Experimenal Child Psychology*, 5, pp. 303–17.

Evans, R.W., Allardyce, R.A., Fergusson, D.M. and Taylor, E. (1981), 'Maternal diet and infantile colic in breast-fed infants', *Lancet*, 1, pp. 1340–2.

Farran, C. and Farran, D. (1981), 'The screaming baby blues', *Parents*, July, pp. 56–60.

Field, T., Ignatoff, E., Stringer, S., Brennan, J., Greenberg, R., Windmayer, S. and Anderson, G.C. (1982), 'Nonnutritive sucking during tube feedings: effects on preterm neonates in an intensive care unit', *Pediatrics*, 70, pp. 381–4.

Forsyth, B.W.C. (1989), 'Colic and the effect of changing milk formulas: a double-blind, multiple-crossover study', *Journal of Pediatrics*, 115, pp. 521–6.

Forsyth, B.W.C. and Canny, P.F. (1991), 'Perceptions of vulnerability $3\frac{1}{2}$ years after problems of feeding and crying behavior in early infancy', *Pediatrics*, 88, pp. 757–63.

Forsyth, B.W.C., Leventhal, J.M. and McCarthy, P.L. (1985a), 'Mothers' perceptions of problems of feeding and crying behaviors: a prospective study', *American Journal of Disease in Childhood*, 139, pp. 269–72.

Forsyth, B.W.C., McCarthy, P.L. and Leventhal, J.M. (1985b), 'Problems of early infancy, formula changes, and mothers' beliefs about their infants', *Journal of Pediatrics*, 106, pp. 1012–17.

Frodi, A. (1985), 'When empathy fails: aversive infant crying and child abuse', in B.M. Lester and C.F. Boukydis (eds), *Infant Crying: Theoretical and research perspectives* (New York: Plenum), pp. 263–78.

Frodi, A. and Lamb, M.E. (1980), 'Child abusers' responses to infant smiles and cries', *Child Development*, 51, pp. 238–41.

Gill, L. (1987), 'Cry baby blues', *The Times*, 26 February, p. 9.

Grunseit, F. (1977), 'Evaluation of the efficacy of dicyclomine hydrochloride (Merbentyl) syrup in the treatment of infant colic', *Current Medical Research Opinion*, 5, pp. 258–61.

Hewson, P., Oberklaid, F. and Menahem, S. (1987), 'Infant colic, distress, and crying', *Clinical Pediatrics*, 26, pp. 69–75.

Hill, S.M. and Milla, P.J. (1990), 'Colitis caused by food allergy in infants', *Archives of Disease in Childhood*, 65, pp. 132–40.

Hubbard, F.O.A. and van Ijzendoorn, M.H. (1991), 'Maternal unresponsiveness and infant crying across the first 9 months: a naturalistic longitudinal study', *Infant Behavior and Development*, 14, pp. 299–312.

Hunziker, U. (1990), 'Der Einfluß des Tragens auf das Schreiverhalten des Säuglings', in M.J. Pachler and H.M. Strassburg (eds), *Der unruhige Säugling* (Hamburg: Hansischer Buchverlag), pp. 235–41.

Hunziker, U.A. and Barr, R.G. (1986), 'Increased carrying reduces infant crying: a randomized controlled trial', *Pediatrics*, 77, pp. 641–8.

Hwang, C.P. and Danielsson, B. (1985), 'Dicyclomine hydrochloride in infantile colic', *British Medical Journal*, 291, p. 1041.

Iacono, G., Carrocio, A., Montalto, G., Gavataio, F., Bragion, E., Lorello, D., Balsamo, V. and Notarbartolo, A. (1991), 'Severe infantile colic and food intolerance: a long-term prospective study', *Journal of Pediatric Gastroenterology and Nutrition*, 12, pp. 332–5.

Illingworth R.S. (1959), 'Evening colic in infants. A double blind trial of dicyclomine hydrochloride', *Lancet*, 2, pp. 119–20.

Illingworth, R.S. (1985), 'Infantile colic revisited', *Archives of Disease in Childhood*, 60, pp. 981–5.

Jackson, H. and Rawlins, M.D. (1977), 'The sleepless child', *British Medical Journal*, 2, p. 509.

Jakobsson, I. and Lindberg, T. (1978), 'Cow's milk as a cause of infantile colic in breast-fed infants', *Lancet*, 2, pp. 437–9.

Jakobsson, I. and Lindberg, T. (1983), 'Cow's milk proteins cause infantile colic in breast-fed infants: a double-blind crossover study', *Pediatrics*, 71, pp. 268–71.

Jenkins, S., Owen, C., Bax, M. and Hart, H. (1984), 'Continuities of common behaviour problems in preschool children', *Journal of Child Psychology and Psychiatry*, 25, pp. 75–89.

Karoly, P. (1980), 'Operant methods', in F.H. Kanfer and A.P. Goldstein (eds), *Helping People Change* (Oxford: Pergamon), pp. 210–47.

Kirkland, J. (1979), 'Child abuse: the crying baby at risk', in A. Neale and R. Renwick (eds), *Early Childhood in New Zealand: Their needs – our concern, Proceedings of Second Early Childhood Convention*, Christchurch, New Zealand, August.

Klougart, N., Nilsson, N. and Jacobsen, J. (1989), 'Infantile colic treated by chiropractors: a prospective study of 316 cases', *Journal of Manipulative and Physiological Therapeutics*, 12, pp. 281–8.

Korner, A.F., Schneider, P. and Forrest, T. (1983), 'Effects of vestibular-proprioceptive stimulation on the neurobehavioral development of preterm infants: a pilot study', *Neuropediatrics*, 14, pp. 170–5.

Larson, K. and Ayllon, T. (1990), 'The effects of contingent music and differential reinforcement on infantile colic', *Behaviour Research and Therapy*, 28, pp. 119–25.

Lester, B.M., Garcia-Coll, C.T. and Valcarcel, M. (1989), 'Perception of infant cries in adolescent and adult mothers', *Journal of Youth and Adolescence*, 18, pp. 231–43.

Levine, M.I. and Bell, A.I. (1950), 'The treatment of "colic" in infancy by use of pacifier', *Journal of Pediatrics*, 37, pp. 750–5.

Lewis, M. (1992), 'Self knowledge and social development in early life', in L.A. Pervin (ed.), *Handbook of Social Psychology* (New York: Guilford) in press.

Liebman, W.M. (1981), 'Infantile colic. Association with lactose and milk intolerance', *Journal of the American Medical Association*, 245, pp. 732–7.

Lipton, E.L., Steinschneider, A. and Richmond, J.B. (1965), 'Swaddling, a child care practice: historical, cultural and experimental observations', *Pediatrics*, 34, pp. 521–67.

Lothe, L. and Lindberg, T. (1989), 'Cow's milk whey protein elicits symptoms of infantile colic in colicky formula-fed infants: a double blind crossover study', *Pediatrics*, 83, pp. 262–6.

Lothe, L., Lindberg, T. and Jakobsson, I. (1982), 'Cow's milk formula as a cause of infantile colic: a double blind study', *Pediatrics*, 70, pp. 7–10.

Lounsbury, M.L. and Bates, J.E. (1982), 'The cries of infants of differing levels of perceived temperamental difficultness: acoustic properties and effects on listeners', *Child Development*, 53, pp. 677–86.

McDevitt, S.C. (1986), 'Continuity and discontinuity of temperament in infancy and early childhood: a psychometric perspective', in R. Plomin and J. Dunn (eds), *The Study of Temperament: Changes, continuities and challenges* (Hillsdale, NJ: Lawrence Erlbaum).

McKenzie, S.A. (1991), 'Troublesome crying in infants: the effect of advice to reduce stimulation', *Archives of Disease in Childhood*, 66, pp. 1416–20.

Merrett, T.G., Burr, M.L., Butland, B.K., Merrett, J. and Vaughan-Williams, E. (1988), '12-month prospective study of 500 babies born into allergic families', *Annals of Allergy*, 61, pp. 13–20.

Messer, D. and Richards, M. (1993), 'The development of sleeping difficulties', in I. St. James-Roberts, G. Harris and D. Messer (eds), *Infant Crying, Feeding and Sleeping: Development, problems and interventions* (Hemel Hempstead: Harvester Wheatsheaf), pp. 150–73.

Miller, A.R. and Barr, R.G. (1991), 'Infantile colic: is it a gut issue?', *Pediatric Clinics of North America*, 38, pp. 1407–23.

Miskelly, F.G., Burr, M.L., Vaughan-Williams, E., Fehly, A.M., Butland, B.K. and Merrett, T.G. (1988), 'Infant feeding and allergy', *Archives of Disease in Childhood*, 63, pp. 388–93.

Moore, T. and Ucko, L.E. (1957), 'Night waking in early infancy', *Archives of Disease in Childhood*, 32, pp. 333–42.

Murooka, H., Tsutoma, A., Tsuyoshi, S., Yusuo, I., Mitsukazu, N. and Nobuhiro, S. (1975), 'Induction of rest and sleep in the neonates by the rhythm of the maternal blood flow', *Nippon Ika Daigaku Zasshi*, 42, pp. 77–9.

Murray, B. and Campbell, D. (1971), 'Sleep states in the newborn: influence of sound', *Neuropädiatrie*, 2, pp. 335–42.

Papousek, M. (1985), 'Umgang mit dem schreienden Säugling und sozialpädiatrische Beratung', *Sozialpädiatrie*, 7, pp. 294–300.

Paradise, J.L. (1966), 'Maternal and other factors in the etiology of infantile colic. Report of a prospective study of 146 infants', *Journal of the American Medical Association*, 197, pp. 123–99.

Parker, S.J. and Barrett, D.E. (1992), 'Maternal type A behavior during pregnancy, neonatal crying, and early infant temperament: do type A women have type A babies?', *Pediatrics*, 89, pp. 474–9.

Pederson, D.R. (1975), 'The soothing effects of rocking as determined by the direction and frequency of movement', *Canadian Journal of Behavioral Sciences*, 7, pp. 237–43.

Pederson, D.R. and Ter Vrught, D. (1973), 'The influence of amplitude and frequency of vestibular stimulation on the activity of two-month-old infants', *Child Development*, 44, pp. 122–8.

Pridham, K.F., Knight, C.B. and Stephenson, G.R. (1989), 'Mothers' working models of infant feeding: description and influencing factors', *Journal of Advanced Nursing*, 14, pp. 1051–61.

Pritchard, P. (1986), 'An infant crying clinic', *Health Visitor*, 59, pp. 375–7.

Rubin, S.P. and Prendergast, M. (1984), 'Infantile colic: incidence and treatment in a Norfolk community', *Child: Care, Health and Development*, 10, pp. 219–26.

St. James-Roberts, I. (1992), 'Managing infants who cry persistently', *British Medical Journal*, 304, pp. 997–8.

St. James-Roberts, I. (1993), in I. St. James-Roberts, G. Harris and D. Messer (eds), *Infant Crying, Feeding and Sleeping: Development, problems and interventions* (Hemel Hempstead: Harvester Wheatsheaf, pp. 26–46.

St. James-Roberts, I. and Halil, T. (1991), 'Infant crying patterns in the first year: normative and clinical findings', *Journal of Child Psychology and Psychiatry*, 32 pp. 951–68.

St. James-Roberts, I., Hurry, J., Bowyer, J. (1992a), 'Objective confirmation of crying levels in infants referred for excessive crying', *Archives of Disease in Childhood*, in press.

St. James-Roberts, I., Hurry, J., Bowyer, J. and Barr, R.G. (1992b), submitted.

St. James-Roberts, I. and Wolke, D. (1988), 'Convergences and discrepancies among mothers' and professionals' assessments of difficult neonatal behaviour', *Journal of Child Psychology and Psychiatry*, 29, pp. 21–42.

St. James-Roberts, I. and Wolke, D. (1989), 'Do obstetric factors affect the mother's perception of her new-born's behaviour?', *British Journal of Developmental Psychology*, 7, pp. 141–58.

Salk, L. (1962), 'Mother's heartbeat as an imprinting stimulus', *Transactions of the New York Academy of Sciences*, 24, p. 753.

Sampson, H.A. (1989), 'Infantile colic and food allergy: fact or fiction?', *Journal of Pediatrics*, 115, pp. 583–4.

Sander, L.W. (1969), 'Comments on regulation and organization in the early infant–caregiver system', in R.J. Robinson (ed.), *Brain and Early Behavior* (New York: Academic).

Sander, L.W. (1987), 'Awareness of inner experience: a systems perspective on self-regulation process in early development', *Child Abuse and Neglect*, 11, pp. 339–46.

Schieffenhövel, W. (1990), 'Ethnologisch-humanethologische Beobachtungen zur Interaktion mit Säuglingen', in M.J. Pachler and H.M. Strassburg (eds), *Der unruhige Säugling* (Hamburg: Hansischer Buchverlag), pp. 25–40.

Schmitt, B.D. (1985), 'Colic: excessive crying in newborns', *Clinics of Perinatology*, 12, pp. 441–51.

Schmitt, B.D. (1986), 'The prevention of sleep problems and colic', *Pediatric Clinics of North America*, 33, pp. 763–74.

Schölmerich, A. and Hwang, P. (1991), 'Exzessives Schreien bei Säuglingen: Verlaufs-merkmale über 15 Monate und Wahrnehmung des Säuglings durch die Eltern', Poster auf der Tagung der Fachgruppe Entwicklungspsychologie in der Deutschen Gesellschaft für Psychologie, Köln, September.

Scott, G. and Richards, M.P.M. (1990), 'Night waking in infants: effects of providing advice and support for parents', *Journal of Child Psychology and Psychiatry*, 31, pp. 551–67.

Shannon, W.R. (1921), 'Colic in breast-fed infants as a result of sensitization to foods in the mother's dietary', *Archives of Paediatrics*, **38**, pp. 756–61.

Shaw, C. (1977), 'A comparison of the patterns of mother–baby interaction for a group of crying, irritable babies and a group of more amenable babies', *Child: Care, Health and Development*, **3**, pp. 1–12.

Skuse, D. and Wolke, D. (1992), 'The nature and consequences of feeding problems in infants', in P. Cooper and A. Stein (eds), *The Nature and Management of Feeding Problems and Eating Disorders in Young People* (New York: Hardwood), pp. 1–25.

Skuse, D., Wolke, D. and Reilly, S. (1991), 'Failure to thrive. Clinical and developmental aspects', in H. Remschmidt and M. Schmidt (eds), *Child and Young Psychiatry, European Perspectives, Vol. II, Developmental Psychopathology* (Bern: Hans Huber).

Smith, C.R. and Steinschneider, A. (1975), 'Differential effects of prenatal rhythmic stimulation on neonatal arousal states', *Child Development*, **46**, pp. 574–8.

Snow, M.E., Jacklin, C.N. and Maccoby, E.E. (1980), 'Crying episodes and sleep–wakefulness transitions in the first 26 months of life', *Infant Behavior and Development*, **3**, pp. 387–94.

Solomon, R.L. and Lessac, M.S.A. (1968), 'A control design for experimental studies of developmental processes', *Psychological Bulletin*, **70**, pp. 145–50.

Sosland, J.M. and Christophersen, E.R. (1991), 'Does SleepTight work? A behavioral analysis of the effectiveness of SleepTight for the management of infant colic', *Journal of Applied Behavioral Analysis*, **24**, pp. 161–6.

Spencer, J.A.D., Moran, D.J., Lee, A. and Talbert, D. (1990), 'White noise and sleep induction', *Archives of Disease in Childhood*, **65**, pp. 135–7.

Stahlberg, M.R. and Savilahti, E. (1986), 'Infantile colic and feeding', *Archives of Disease in Childhood*, **61**, pp. 1232–3.

Stores, G. (1990), 'Sleep disorders in children', *British Medical Journal*, **301**, pp. 351–2.

Taitz, L.S. (1982), 'Soy feeding in infancy', *Archives of Disease in Childhood*, **57**, pp. 814–15.

Taitz, L.S. and Wardley, B.L. (1989), *Handbook of Child Nutrition* (Oxford: Oxford University Press).

Taubman, B. (1984), 'Clinical trial of the treatment of colic by modification of parent–infant interaction', *Pediatrics*, **74**, pp. 995–1003.

Taubman, B. (1988), 'Parental counselling compared with elimination of cow's milk or soy milk protein for the treatment of infant colic syndrome: a randomized trial', *Pediatrics*, **81**, pp. 756–61.

Ter Vrught, D. and Pederson, D.R. (1973), 'The effects of vertical rocking frequencies in the arousal level in two-month-old infants', *Child Development*, **44**, pp. 205–9.

Trevathen, C. (1987), 'Sharing makes sense: intersubjectivity and the making of an infant's meaning', in R. Steele and T. Threadgold (eds), *Language Topics Essays in Honor of Michael Halliday. Vol. 1* (Philadelphia: John Benjamins), pp. 177–99.

van den Boom, D. (1988), 'Neonatal irritability and the development of attachment: observation and intervention', PhD Dissertation, University of Leiden, The Netherlands.

van den Daele, L. (1970), 'Modification of infant state by treatment in a rockerbox', *Journal of Psychology*, **74**, pp. 161–5.

Vandenplas, Y., Deneyer, M., Sacre, L. and Loeb, H. (1988), 'Preliminary data on a field study with a new hypo-allergic formula', *European Journal of Paediatrics*, **148**, pp. 274–7.

Vaughn, B.E., Joffe, L.S., Bradley, C.F., Seifer, R. and Barglow, P. (1987), 'Maternal characteristics measured prenatally are predictive of rating of temperamental "difficulty" on the Carey Infant Temperament Questionnaire', *Developmental Psychology*, 23, pp. 152–61.

Warner, J.O. and Hathaway, M.J. (1984), 'Allergic form of Meadow's syndrome (Munchausen by proxy)', *Archives of Disease in Childhood*, 59, pp. 151–6.

Weissbluth, M., Christoffel, K.K. and Davis, A.T. (1984), 'Treatment of infantile colic with dicyclomine hydrochloride', *Journal of Pediatrics*, 104, pp. 951–5.

Wessel, M.A., Cobb, J.C., Jackson, E.B., Harris, G.S. and Detwiler, A.C. (1954), 'Paroxysmal fussing in infancy, sometimes called "colic"', *Pediatrics*, 14, pp. 421–35.

Wiesenfeld, A.R., Malatesta, C.Z. and DeLoach, L.L. (1981), 'Differential parental response to familiar and unfamiliar infant distress signals', *Infant Behavior and Development*, 4, pp. 281–95.

Williams, C.D. (1959), 'The elimination of tantrum behavior by an extinction procedure', *Journal of Abnormal and Social Psychology*, 59, p. 269.

Wolff, P.H. (1987), *The Development of Behavioral States and the Expression of Emotions in Early Infancy: New proposals for investigation* (Chicago: University of Chicago Press).

Wolke, D. (1986), 'The screaming baby: Anmerkungen zu dem Beitrag von Mangold und Fuchs', *Pädiatrie und Pädiologie*, 21, pp. 367–76.

Wolke, D. (1988), 'What is a screaming baby?', Paper presented at the Annual Conference of the Developmental Psychology Section of the British Psychological Society, Harlech, Wales.

Wolke, D. (1990), 'Schwierige Säuglinge: Wirklichkeit oder Einbildung?', in M.J. Pachler, and H.M. Strassburg (eds), *Der unruhige Säugling* (Hamburg: Hansischer Buchverlag), pp. 70–88.

Wolke, D. (1991a), 'Supporting the preterm baby's psychological development', annotation, *Journal of Child Psychology and Psychiatry*, 32, pp. 723–41.

Wolke, D. (1991b), 'Psycho-biologische Aspekte der Pflege von Frühgeborenen', *Deutsche Krankenpflege-Zeitschrift*, 44, pp. 478–83.

Wolke, D. (1993a), 'Feeding and sleeping', in M. Rutter and D. Hay (eds), *Developmental Principles and Clinical Issues in Psychology and Psychiatry* (Oxford: Blackwell), in press.

Wolke, D. (1993b), 'Die Entwichlung und Behandlung von Schlafproblemen und excessivem schreien', in F. Petermann (ed.), *Verhaltenstherapie mit Kindern* (München: Röttger Verlag), pp. 145–99.

Wolke, D. and Eldridge, T. (1992), 'Environmental care', in A.G.M. Campbell and N. McIntosh (eds), *Forfar & Arneil's Textbook of Paediatrics*, 4th edn (London: Churchill Livingstone).

Wolke, D. and Gray, P. (1989), 'Helping parents cope with their screaming baby: a controlled treatment study', Presentation at the 4th World Congress for Infant Psychiatry and Allied Disciplines, Lugano, Switzerland, 20–24 September.

Wolke, D., Gray, P. and Meyer, R. (1993a), 'Validity of the Crying Pattern Questionnaire: a research note', *Journal of Reproductive and Infant Psychology*, in press.

Wolke, D., Gray, P. and Meyer, R. (1993b), 'Excessive infant crying: A controlled study of mothers helping mothers', *Pediatrics*, in press.

Wolke, D. and St. James-Roberts, I. (1986), 'Maternal affective-cognitive processes in the perception of newborn difficultness', in G.A. Kohnstamm (ed.), *Temperament Discussed* (Lisse: Swets and Zeitlinger B.V.), pp. 27–34.

Wolke, D. and St. James-Roberts, I. (1987), 'Multi-method measurement of the early parent–infant system with easy and difficult newborns', in H. Rauh and H.C.

Steinhausen (eds), *Psychobiology and Early Development* (Oxford: North-Holland), pp. 49–70.

Wolke, D. and Skuse, D. (1992), 'The management of infant feeding problems', in P. Cooper and A. Stein (eds), *The Nature and Management of Feeding Problems and Eating Disorders in Young People* (New York: Hardwood).

Wright, P. (1989), 'Feeding experiences in early infancy', in R. Shepherd (ed.), *Handbook of the Psychophysiology of Human Eating* (Chichester: Wiley), pp. 157–78.

Zuckerman, B., Bauchner, H., Parker, S. and Cabral, H. (1990), 'Maternal depressive symptoms during pregnancy, and newborn irritability', *Journal of Developmental and Behavioral Pediatrics*, 11, pp. 190–4.

Part 2

Feeding

Chapter 4

The infant's regulation of nutritional intake

R.F. Drewett, *University of Durham*

Introduction

It is always a temptation to think that infants are rather simple, but in relation to their regulation of nutritional intake there are at least three complexities that we do not find in adults. First, the natural adaptation of the human infant is to breast-feeding. This involves interactions with the mother which are physiological as well as behavioural and which affect the supply of milk as well as its consumption. Second, milk intake in infants serves to provide both food and water. When we consider nutritional intake we need to remember that there may be complex possibilities of cross-stimulation or cross-satiation between the hunger and thirst systems, assuming (it is open to question) that these systems are present from birth in the same form as they are found later in adults. Third, infants, unlike adults, grow. There is good evidence that their growth is regulated or 'target-seeking': it is very regular, and when growth velocity is reduced due to childhood illnesses it subsequently increases during catch-up growth (Tanner, 1986). So in infants the regulation of intake needs to be considered in relation to expected height for age, as well as to expected weight for height. Regulation is about a set trajectory, rather than a set point. Of course, the fact that an infant has to learn a completely different way of taking in food and water half-way through the first year, when weaning begins, adds yet another complexity, but I shall be concentrating in this chapter on early infancy, mainly because there has been so little systematic research on the behavioural aspects of weaning.

Energy balance

It is often a tacit assumption of nutritional thinking that if the milk intake of an infant is adequate to meet energy requirements, it would be adequate to meet protein requirements (Whitehead *et al.*, 1982). Evidence that the assumption is well founded is provided by Waterlow and Thomson (1979). If it is, the separate regulation of protein intake would be unnecessary in infants, and a simplifying assumption would be that the regulation of nutritional intake in milk-fed infants would just involve the regulation of energy intake.

The infant's task is to ensure that its intake is sufficient to satisfy its needs. Energy is deposited as new tissue during growth, or expended – for basal metabolism, thermogenesis, the energy cost of tissue synthesis and for activity. The energy deposited as new tissue can be calculated from studies of body composition (see, for example, Fomon *et al.*, 1988), and total energy expenditure can be measured using the doubly labelled water method (Coward, 1988). Immediately after birth a substantial proportion of energy needs are for growth (about a third, Prentice *et al.*, 1988). This proportion drops very rapidly, with the falling growth velocity of the infant, to 2–3 per cent by one year of age. Most of the energy needed by the older infant, therefore, is for expenditure rather than growth. How much of the expended energy is used for activity is harder to answer. Basal metabolic rate can be estimated, and suggestions have been made for the energy 'costing' of different activities (e.g. 1.2, 1.5 and 2 times BMR for lying, sitting and standing, respectively, and 3.5 times for walking and running: FAO/WHO/UNU, 1985). Measures of time spent in different activities derived from direct observation can then be combined with these costs to give estimates of the energy needs of activity (Vasquez-Velasquez, 1988; Lawrence *et al.*, 1991).

It is these needs for energy for growth and expenditure that the infant must translate into energy intakes, if intakes are to be appropriate. Measured energy intakes in infants over the first year are summarised for a wide range of data sets from Canada, Sweden, the United Kingdom and the United States in Whitehead *et al.* (1982). Mean intakes rise in a linear way with age; for boys, energy (kcal/day) = 456 + 49 (months); for girls, energy = 404 + 49 (months).[1] Expressed in relation to body weight, there is some evidence that energy requirements decline over the first 6–8 months of life and then start increasing again. The decline is due to declining growth velocity, the increase to increased activity. Estimates given by Beaton (1985) suggest a reduction from 124 kcal/kg/day to 94.5 at 8 months, rising to 104.5 at 12 months. Estimates in Whitehead, Paul and Cole (1982) suggest a reduction from 110 to 85 kcal/kg/day over the first six months, rising to 105 at one year; a more recent estimate from the same group, however, suggests only a very small rise, to 85 kcal/kg/day at three years after a drop from 85 at six months to 83 at one year (Prentice *et al.*, 1988).

It is important to appreciate that energy 'requirements', as they are specified in the nutritional literature, are sometimes estimated from measurements of energy storage and expenditure, and sometimes from measurements of energy intake. It is the relationship between energy intake and energy requirements as estimated in the first way (as, for example, in Waterlow and

Thomson, 1979) that shows that infants are regulating in accordance with energy needs. It is also important to appreciate what is meant by energy 'requirements' here. They are the average requirements of infants in a population, if the population is to grow on average like a reference population – for example, like the population upon which the United States National Center for Health Statistics based the growth charts which the World Health Organization recommended for use as an international reference (World Health Organization, 1983). Individual babies, of course, have different individual rates of energy expenditure: centiles are provided by Davies *et al.* (1989), and imply that energy expenditure for a two-month-old baby varies by a factor of about two between infants on the 10th centile (expenditure about 1000 kJ/day) and those on the 90th (about 2000 kJ/day). Finally, it is important to appreciate that energy requirements are themselves open to regulation to some extent, via the regulation of energy expenditure (Keesey and Powley, 1986).

Feeding behaviour

The regulation of the intake of an infant is achieved by the mother–infant pair, not by the infant acting in isolation. The interactions between the mother and infant are complex, and in breast-fed infants are physiological as well as behavioural. Maternal hormones released in response to sucking, prolactin from the anterior pituitary gland and oxytocin from the posterior pituitary gland are responsible both for milk synthesis and for milk flow.

It is obvious enough that infants alternate between a sleeping and a waking state, with feeding restricted to the waking state. Less obvious is whether the state changes are themselves hunger dependent: we have little systematically collected data, for example, on the relationship between the size of a feed and the length of the succeeding sleep. Matheny *et al.* (1990) examined the relationship between milk consumed at feeds and the intervals to the next feed (the 'postprandial' intervals). These would include time spent sleeping, but not be restricted to it. The most striking feature of the results was their variation from infant to infant: the range across infants in the correlation between meal size and the postprandial interval at two weeks, for example, was −0.29 to 0.62; at six weeks it was −0.53 to 0.24 and at twelve weeks −0.63 to 0.73. Macknin *et al.* (1989) examined the effect of adding rice cereal to bottle feeds given last thing at night, in a well-designed study with the infants randomly assigned to a supplemented and an unsupplemented group. The supplement had no clear effect on sleeping through the night. Although the question could usefully have more systematic investigation, at the moment there is no good reason to think that time spent sleeping forms part of the regulation of food intake in infants.

When the infant is awake, hunger can be signalled using crying (a non-specific signal) and, given appropriate responses by the mother, feeding initiated using behaviour patterns specific to feeding. The first of these is the 'directed head turning response' or 'rooting reflex' which was studied in detail by Prechtl (1958). He provides evidence that milk intake inhibits this response for several hours. The study is presented in a rather informal way: it is not clear whether the amount of milk fed to the infant was controlled experimentally or left free to vary naturally, and results from unfed controls are only referred to incidentally. But the data provided do suggest that directed head turning responses could be developed into at least a semi-quantitative measure of hunger that could be used equally well in bottle- and in breast-fed babies.

Sucking rates in human infants vary with the rate of milk flow, becoming faster as milk flow decreases (Wolff, 1968; Bowen-Jones *et al.*, 1982). There is some uncertainty as to whether the variation in sucking is continuous or discontinuous.Wolff argued that infants switch between two types of sucking, with different patterning and modal rates. However, in a study using precise measurement of intersuck intervals by means of an intra-oral cannula there was no evidence that sucking rates on the breast were bimodal (Woolridge and Drewett, 1986). The rate and patterning of sucking respond to milk flow, and so they cannot be used in any simple way as measures of hunger (see Chapter 5 by Peter Wright, who also discusses satiety signals). There is, however, evidence that in some situations characteristics of sucking do relate to subsequent adiposity (see below).

Milk intake over a feed can be measured accurately, in breast-fed as well as bottle-fed infants, using programmable electronic balances (Drewett *et al.*, 1984). These average over time, allowing weighing accurate to within about 1 g. (It is important not to confuse the actual precision of a balance in use with its nominal precision. Much of the error in weighing infants is due to their movement, especially if they are hungry. The actual precision of a balance in use is generally less than its nominal precision, and can only be determined by replicate weighings.) Test weighing over a 24-hour period provides an estimate of daily intake: daily intake cannot be determined by doubling intake over 12 hours, and it is generally desirable to test weigh over 48 hours to allow an estimate to be made of day-to-day variation.

It is milk intake that the infant must regulate to control its energy intake, but it is important to remember that the functional capacity of the breast also varies from mother to mother (Hytten, 1954). Low intake may in theory be attributable either to a lack of hunger in the infant or to the mother's milk-producing capacity being low, and there is evidence that the explanation is different in different mother–infant pairs (Dewey and Lonnerdal, 1986). If the baby is bottle-fed, variation attributable to the mother's milk supply is eliminated. While this can be useful experimentally, it also eliminates part of the natural regulatory system, which involves the mother's response to sucking (prolactin release and milk synthesis) as well as the infant's behaviour.

Regulation of energy intake

If energy intake is regulated by infants, the volume of milk taken would be expected to vary (a) inversely with variations in its energy content, and (b) directly with variations in the baby's energy needs.

When feeds are of the same energy density, it makes no difference to the energy intake of the infant whether the energy is present as fat or carbohydrate. This was shown by Fomon *et al.* (1976), who compared intake of two formulas. In one, 29 per cent of the calories were present as fat and 62 per cent as carbohydrate; in the other, 57 per cent were present as fat and 34 per cent as carbohydrate. The energy intake of infants fed on the two formulas was the same. This is one piece of evidence in favour of the view that it is energy that infants are regulating.

Fomon *et al.* (1969) also compared the intake of male infants fed by bottle from two different formulas similar except for water content. One provided 0.67 kcal/ml, which approximates to standard formula and to breast milk, and the other provided 1.33 kcal/ml. The infants fed the more concentrated formula took in less milk, as one would expect if energy intake was being regulated. But in the first 42 days the reduction was not enough to compensate for its increased energy density, so intake in calories increased.

Hunt (1980) suggests that these results can be explained on the basis of known properties of the duodenal receptors that regulate gastric emptying. The regulation of gastric emptying is inhibitory. When food contains fats or carbohydrate, gastric emptying rate is slowed as a result of stimulation of two different sets of duodenal receptor. One responds to osmotic stimulation, and so slows gastric emptying when the food contains sugars or carbohydrates, since these are broken down into monosaccharides. The other responds to fatty acid anions produced by the digestion of fats. Although the two sets of receptors are independent, they are 'tuned' so that equal calories slow gastric emptying by the same amount, whether the calories are derived from carbohydrates or fats (Hunt and Stubbs, 1975). Hunt (1980) shows that the relationship between the energy density of a meal (x, kcal/ml) and the calories emptying from the stomach in 30 minutes (y, kcal/30 mins) is $y = 56 + 85.4x$. The implication can be seen by comparing, for example, a meal of 150 kcal fed at energy densities of either 0.65 kcal/ml or 0.87 kcal/ml. After 30 minutes 75 per cent of the first meal will have left the stomach (112 kcal) compared with 87 per cent of the second meal (130 kcal).

Hunt proposes that the infant's milk intake responds in the same way as gastric emptying, implying that (a) it would make no difference to intake whether calories in the milk were derived from carbohydrate or fat, and (b) increasing the calorific content of food would reduce intake not by an amount sufficient to maintain calorie intake constant, but by an amount predictable from the change in gastric emptying rate.

The first prediction was exactly met in Fomon *et al.*'s results, as noted above. The second was also approximately met. For the data given in Fomon *et al.* (1969), the approximation is not actually a very good one. Formulas of 0.67 and 1.33 kcal/ml were compared. Using the regression equation given above to determine changes in gastric emptying rate, the 'predicted' change in intake in calories when infants are fed the more rather than the less concentrated formula is therefore 100 (170−113)/113 = 50 per cent. The measured change in intake was 32 per cent.

The approximation is much better using formulas that differ less extremely from breast-milk. Fomon *et al.* (1975) compared the intake of infants fed a formula providing 0.54 kcal/ml and those fed a formula providing 1.00 kcal/ml. When x is changed from 0.54 to 1.0, the predicted difference in intake in calories is 100(141−102)/102 = 38 per cent. The measured intakes for the two groups over the first six weeks were 393 and 538 kcal/day, respectively, a difference of 37 per cent.

Further sets of data of a similar kind have since been published by Brooke and Kinsey (1985) and by Lucas *et al.* (1992). In the first study seventeen low-birth-weight infants were randomly assigned to two groups, and fed either 0.65 kcal/ml or 0.87 kcal/ml. On Hunt's model this gives a predicted difference in intake in calories of 17 per cent. The actual intakes at six weeks were 484 and 555 kcal/day, a difference of 15 per cent. In the second study 32 preterm infants were randomly assigned to feeds of 0.72 or 0.68 kcal/ml. Over the first three months average intake of the higher calorie feed was 3 per cent higher than intake of the lower calorie feed; the predicted increase is 2 per cent.

These papers show that increased energy density in milk is only partly compensated for by reduced intake in the early weeks of life, and that the extent of the increased energy intake can be predicted from the effect of energy-yielding substances on gastric emptying rate. Hunt notes that this could be a coincidence, and there is certainly an element of arbitrariness in using emptying over 30 minutes to predict intake. What seems reasonably certain, however, is the implication that in these very young infants it is not the total intake of calories summed over 24 hours that is regulating milk intake, but some more local signal responsive to calories leaving the stomach or small intestine. A fixed number of calories leave the gut more rapidly if they are given in a denser form, and so total intake goes up as a result.

Fomon *et al.* went on to show that by about six weeks of age the energy intakes of infants fed the two formulas were not significantly different – the infants fed the high calorie formula were compensating entirely for its greater energy density. This change is unlikely to be due to developmental changes in gastric emptying mechanisms, since the properties assumed for them by Hunt are all based on generalisations from adults. It is more likely that the infant is developing a system for monitoring its energy intake that is relatively independent of local gastric emptying rates.

So far we have been concerned with regulation in relation to changes in dietary energy density. A different and more difficult question is how energy intake in infants is regulated in relation to their energy needs. Here we have a problem that is more complex in the infant than the adult: in the adult growth has stopped, and regulation can therefore be thought of as regulation about a set point. In the infant we need to think of a 'set trajectory' rather than a set point.

Ounsted and Sleigh (1975), in a paper entitled 'The infant's self-regulation of food intake and weight gain' argued that small-for-dates infants 'actively counteract the effects of their slow growth in utero by regulating their food intake after birth. The same applies, in the reverse direction, to large-for-dates infants'. The data on which their argument is based come from a comparison of normal controls with a sample born to hypertensive mothers and a small-for-dates and large-for-dates sample. In these infants milk intake expressed as ml per kg body weight was negatively correlated with body weight at two months.

The difficulty here is that there was in fact no significant difference in milk intake between the four groups, which makes milk intake effectively a constant. It follows that there is bound to be a negative correlation between milk intake divided by body weight and body weight itself, but the same would be true using any other constant. The result reported by Ounsted and Sleigh is compatible with the view that intake in the infant is precisely regulated to meet its needs for growth, but it is equally compatible with the view that no behavioural regulation is operating at all. Even if no behavioural regulation were operating at all, there would still be an effect on growth that would look as if it were self-regulatory, deriving from the lower maintenance needs of the smaller infants, which would spare more energy for growth if intake were constant.

Other evidence for behavioural regulation in relation to need in the special case of 'catch-up' growth is provided for slightly older children by Ashworth (1969, 1974). These papers dealt with energy intake during recovery from malnutrition in a group of West Indian children 10–36 months old. They were hospitalised for malnutrition, with weight for height ranging from 53 to 70 per cent of an American (Boston) standard, and were fed on a high-energy milk preparation. There were striking changes in their acceptance of food over time. In the first six weeks growth rate was about fifteen times as fast as that of normal children of the same age, and virtually no food refusal was recorded. At about the time they reached their expected weight for height, six of the eight children abruptly started refusing feeds, and the rates of weight gain then fell off.

Changes in weight for height do not necessarily reflect changes in linear growth, so it is difficult to be sure of the interpretation of this result. It is possible that the infants were indeed regulating their food intake in relation to their expected linear growth, but the alternative that they were regulating the level of their fat stores – or some related variable – cannot be excluded. Indeed, their growth rates were still three times the normal for age after expected weight for height was reached.

There are cases of breast-fed infants who do not grow, and who may even become seriously malnourished, for reasons which must be classed as failures of milk transfer from the mother (Hytten *et al.*, 1958; Davies and Evans, 1976; Gilmore and Rowland, 1978). This may be due to a primary failure of milk production in the mother. There are certainly examples of this; the diagnostic key is a lack of change in breast volume during pregnancy, indicating a lack of growth of alveolar tissue (Neifert *et al.*, 1985). If this can be excluded, one would look for secondary failure attributable to inadequate sucking. This may be a motor problem: some infants do not attach satisfactorily to the nipple, a skill which can be taught. But there is evidence that other babies are content on a level of milk intake that does not provide adequately for growth. Davies and Evans (1976) report a boy whose weight at eight weeks was 220 g below birth weight. He was described by the mother as a contented baby, demanding a feed every 4–5 hr by day and sleeping 12 hr at night, and a slow feeder. Conversely, there are infants whose energy intake is adequate, as shown by adequate growth, but who seem persistently hungry (Yorston and Hytten, 1957).

That an infant's sucking style affects its weight gain is indicated by the results of Pollitt *et al.* (1978) and Agras *et al.* (1987, 1990). Pollitt *et al.* showed that weight gain during the first month of life is predictable from the infant's sucking behaviour on the first or second day of life. The relevant predictor was number of refusals of the nipple by the infant, which correlated −0.33 with weight gain over the first month. Agras *et al.* showed that characteristics of sucking measured during a bottle feed in the first month predicted adiposity at one, two and three years of age, in a sample that was predominantly breast-fed in the first month. The 'vigorous feeding style' which was associated with a higher intake of calories and greater adiposity consisted of sucking 'more rapidly, at higher pressure, with a longer suck and burst duration, and a shorter interval between bursts of sucking'. Follow-up showed that by six years the effect had disappeared; by then parental education was a major predictor, with poorer education associated with greater adiposity. Obesity is not necessarily behavioural in origin, however; differences in energy expenditure are also relevant. Roberts *et al.* (1988) examined energy expenditure and intake in infants born to lean or to overweight mothers. The infants were studied at three months and followed up for the first year. Infants who became overweight by the age of one year did not have a higher food intake at three months, but they did have a lower energy expenditure (about one fifth lower than in those who did not).

There is also an interesting possibility that sucking may affect weight gain independently of its effects on milk intake. The possibility was first raised by Measel and Anderson (1979). Their study showed differences in clinical course when premature infants were given a pacifier during and following tube feeding. Although it was not statistically significant, they also reported a small increase in weight gain (2.6 g/day). Field *et al.* (1982) showed in a randomised trial that infants given a pacifier during tube feedings gained weight faster than those who were not (mean 19.3 g/day versus 16.5 g/day), and Bernbaum *et al.* (1983) reported a similar result (25.7 g/day versus 17.1 g/day). Ernst *et al.* (1989), however, have subsequently found no such effect in a study which controlled more carefully for nutritional intake.

Water balance

The separate regulation of water intake may not generally be a problem for wholly breast-fed infants since water intake is adequately provided for by their milk intake, without any supplementation, even in hot climates (Martines *et al.*, 1992). There are, of course, circumstances in which additional water might be necessary: if renal concentrating ability is impaired, if there is an increased extrarenal loss of fluid, due to diarrhoea for example, or if there is an inappropriate additional intake of protein or salts (Ziegler and Fomon, 1971).

Inappropriately high sodium intake was not uncommon in bottle-fed infants in Great Britain in the 1970s. Taitz and Byers (1972) sampled milk formula feeds brought by mothers with their six- to ten-week-old babies to routine post-natal check-ups. The sodium content of the feeds was 25 per cent higher than in feeds made up correctly, and the mean urinary osmolality of a sample of bottle-fed babies in the clinic was 338 mOsm/kg (range 67 to 1327) as against 105 (43 to 228) in breast-fed infants. A suggestion was often made at that time (e.g. Dunn and Pollnitz, 1975; Morley and Woodland, 1979) that obesity in bottle-fed infants might be accounted for by thirst. The suggestion was that hypertonic feeds stimulated osmotic thirst which led to crying, and this was then misinterpreted by the mother as hunger, leading to further feeds and further osmotic stimulation.

We do not know, however, whether infants do indeed respond to increased plasma osmolality – or to reduced plasma volume – by increasing their intake of milk. The belief that they do so is based on the assumption that the milk intake of infants is regulated like water intake in adults, and on the assumption that infants respond to osmotic thirst stimuli as adults would. The evidence that they do is notable for its absence. The only relevant paper known to me is by Janovsky *et al.* (1967). They loaded breast-fed infants with sodium chloride. Although the load was sufficient to nearly halve the volume of urine the infants produced, there was no evidence for a systematic increase in their milk intake.

Feeding, crying and sleeping

In addition to their normal relationship as part of the daily cycle of behavioural states in infancy, certain problems of crying and sleeping are often thought to be tied up with feeding. Two examples are colicky crying and night waking, and it is to these we now turn.

If the explanation of colic is, indeed, to be found at a gastrointestinal level at all, the most promising candidates at the moment would be incomplete lactose absorption or increased motilin levels.

Incomplete lactose absorption can be detected by the measurement of breath hydrogen, the only known source of which in mammals is the fermentation of carbohydrate by gut bacteria (Ostrander et al., 1983). Barr et al. (1984) found that it was common in the first months of life, and when a group of infants was followed over the first five months, hydrogen excretion increased to a peak in the second month and then dropped from the third month onwards. There is also some evidence of a diurnal rhythm, with peak values in the afternoon. There is some correspondence between these patterns and patterns of crying (St. James-Roberts, 1989), and when infants with colic (inconsolable crying lasting several hours each day for which no clinical cause could be found) were compared with controls, they were found to have significantly higher peak breath hydrogen levels (Miller et al., 1989). The main difficulty is knowing whether colicky crying is an effect of the incomplete absorption of lactose which underlies the increased breath hydrogen levels, or whether colicky crying actually alters their measured values. End-tidal breath hydrogen concentration varies by more than 50 per cent during hyper- or hypoventilation (for example, Bjorneklett and Jenssen, 1980; cited in Ostrander et al., 1983). A longitudinal study is called for to determine the causal sequence underlying this correlation. However, it is worth noting that although Barr et al. (1984) found large differences in breath hydrogen in different behavioural states, they did not find that levels were raised by crying or fussing compared with other states in the same baby: indeed, crying and fussing were associated with lower levels.

A longitudinal study was carried out by Loethe et al. (1990) in their investigation of the relationship between the development of colic and plasma motilin levels. Motilin is a gut hormone, manufactured from cells localised in the duodenum and jejunum, and as its name suggests it has a role in gastric motility. Motilin levels in cord blood, and in venous blood on the first day of life, were significantly higher in infants who subsequently developed colic. The probability of developing colic was about 0.1 in infants with motilin levels below 20 pmol/l on the first day, about 0.2 if they were between 20 and 60, about 0.5 if they were between 60 and 100, and about 1 if they were higher than 100 (calculated from Loethe et al., 1990, Figure 2). Motilin appears to be secreted in response to gastric distension, and to be involved in the control of gastric emptying and the activity of the colon, and it is consistently elevated in diarrhoea (Aynsley-Green, 1989), so this is undoubtedly a promising lead; but it is not clear at the moment how the temporal patterns of colicky crying can be explained by raised motilin levels.

With reference to sleeping, Fagioli et al. (1988) investigated the role of feeding in the development of sleeping rhythms in one of a series of fascinating papers on infants fed parenterally (i.e. by intravenous infusion) from birth.

Twelve infants, six under 3 months old and six 3–12 months old, were compared with twelve controls fed normally. In the parenterally fed infants the feeds were given continuously, day and night. Three sleep states were defined and measured: waking, quiet sleep and paradoxical sleep. The striking finding was that the diurnal rhythm in sleeping that developed over the early months in the normally fed infants developed in exactly the same way in the continuously fed infants, unlike the diurnal rhythm in heart rate, which did not develop in infants fed parenterally (Salzarulo *et al.*, 1980). This suggests that the basic diurnal rhythm in sleep states develops independently of feeding patterns.

There is, however, now good evidence that breast-fed infants are less likely to sleep through the night without a feed than bottle-fed infants. This was shown by Wright *et al.* (1980, 1983), by Eaton-Evans and Dugdale (1988), and by Wailoo *et al.* (1990).

Eaton-Evans and Dugdale cite two results as inconsistent with this generalisation. One of these (Blurton-Jones *et al.*, 1978) appears to be concerned with a rather different issue – the association between sleeping at fifteen months and previous, rather than the current, feeding patterns. The other (Beal, 1969) does report a discrepant result, though no data are given; a second negative result is reported by Macknin *et al.* (1989), incidentally to another study, though again no data are given. At the moment the balance of evidence is in favour of the view that breast-fed infants are more likely to wake in the night; this view is supported by all published studies that present relevant data. Elias *et al.* (1986) have put forward the view that norms for sleeping that show the development of 8 to 10 hours uninterrupted sleep by the age of four months reflect the sleeping patterns of bottle-fed infants. Infants in their sample who were breast-fed for two years continued to wake in the night until they were eventually weaned.

Conclusions

Perhaps I can best conclude by returning to the 'three complexities' with which we began.

The central importance of breast-feeding to maternal and child health internationally derives from its having a double benefit: it both promotes the health of the infant, and delays ovulation in the mother, leading to increased interbirth intervals in populations that do not have easy access to contraceptive methods. Its importance has led to a considerable research tradition in human lactation over the last twenty years, but one that has generally been isolated from any concern with the infant's own motivational regulation. We are just beginning to see this changing. Drewett and Woolridge (1981), for example, showed that during a breast-feed infants 5–7 days old took less milk from the second than the first breast. This was true even when the order was allocated at random, and when any milk lost from the contralateral breast during feeding from the first was weighed and taken into account. It shows that the infants were regulating their own intake and not simply taking all the milk that was available. Dewey *et al.* (1991) have reported that older infants also generally leave milk unconsumed. Tyson *et al.* (1992) have considered the behavioural adaptations shown by babies breast-fed by mothers with low milk fat yields. Complex though the problems are, we need to understand how breast-fed as well as bottle-fed infants regulate their own intake, both because our theoretical understanding of behavioural homeostasis in infants is otherwise seriously incomplete, and because of the practical importance of breast-feeding in relation to infant growth and health.

The motivational specificity of the control of milk intake in infancy is something we know very little about. Although we talk about 'hunger' and 'thirst' in infants it is not clear to what extent the control of sucking and milk intake in infants is in fact the same as the control of food and water intake in adults. In the rat, the only species in which we have a lot of information on behavioural homeostasis both in infants and in adults, a quite good case can be made that the control of sucking and milk intake involves a motivational system *sui generis*, from which the hunger and thirst system take over only at weaning (Drewett, 1978).

The regulation of nutritional intake over the first six months of life is especially interesting because this is the period of very rapid growth. Individual differences in birth weight are mostly environmental in origin, and the correlation between birth length and adult length is only about 0.3; yet by one year the correlation is 0.7, and by two years 0.8 (Roberts, 1981; Tanner, 1981). Catch-up growth is concentrated over the 0–6 month period; catch–down growth over the 3–18 month period (Smith *et al.*, 1976). We are quite ignorant at the moment of the mechanisms by which this relative change in size is achieved, though presumably it must involve a relative adjustment of nutritional intake, implying a complexity in the task underlying motivational regulation in the infant that is wholly absent in the no longer growing adult.

Notes

1. The SI base unit for energy is the joule (J), which generally appears in the nutritional work quoted as the kilojoule (kJ). The calorie (cal) is 4.184 J, and the nutritional calorie (Cal) is 1 kcal or 4.184 kJ. This non-SI unit is also widely used. I have quoted whichever unit appears in the original publication.

References

Agras, W.S., Kraemer, H.C., Berkowitz, R.I. and Hammer, L.D. (1990), 'Influence of early feeding style on adiposity at 6 years of age', *Behavioral Pediatrics*, **116**, pp. 805–9.

Agras, W.S., Kraemer, H.C., Berkowitz, R.I., Korner, A.F. and Hammer, L.D. (1987), 'Does a vigorous feeding style influence early development of adiposity?', *Journal of Pediatrics*, 110, pp. 799–804.

Ashworth, A. (1969), 'Growth rates in children recovering from malnutrition', *British Journal of Nutrition*, 23, pp. 835–45.

Ashworth, A. (1974), 'Ad lib. feeding during recovery from malnutrition', *British Journal of Nutrition*, 31, pp. 109–12.

Aynsley-Green, A. (1989), 'The endocrinology of feeding in the newborn', *Baillières Clinical Endocrinology and Metabolism*, 3, pp. 837–68.

Barr, R.G., Hanley, J., Paterson, D.K. and Wooldridge, J. (1984), 'Breath hydrogen excretion in normal newborn infants in response to usual feeding patterns: evidence for "functional lactase insufficiency" beyond the first month of life', *Journal of Pediatrics*, 104, pp. 527–33.

Beal, V.A. (1969) 'Termination of night feeding in infancy', *Journal of Pediatrics*, 75, pp. 690–2.

Beaton, G.H. (1985), 'Nutritional needs during the first year of life: some concepts and perspectives', *Pediatric Clinics of North America*, 322, pp. 275–88.

Bernbaum, J.C., Pereira, G.R., Watkins, J.B. and Peckham, G.J. (1983), 'Nonnutritive sucking during gavage feeding enhances growth and maturation in premature infants', *Journal of Pediatrics*, 71, pp. 41–5.

Blurton-Jones, N., Ferreira, R., Brown, M.F. and Macdonald, l. (1978), 'The association between perinatal factors and later night waking', *Developmental Medicine and Child Neurology*, 20, pp. 427–34.

Bowen-Jones, A., Thompson, C.T. and Drewett, R.F. (1982), 'Milk flow and sucking rates during breast-feeding', *Developmental Medicine and Child Neurology*, 24, pp. 626–33.

Brooke, O.G. and Kinsey, J.M. (1985), 'High energy feeding in small for gestation infants', *Archives of Disease in Childhood*, 60, pp. 42–6.

Coward, W.A. (1988), 'The $^2H_2$ ^{18}O method – principles and practice', *Proceedings of the Nutrition Society*, 47, pp. 209–18.

Davies, D.P. and Evans, T.I. (1976), 'Failure to thrive at the breast', *Lancet*, 11, pp. 1194–5.

Davies, P.S.W., Ewing, G. and Lucas, A. (1989), 'Energy expenditure in early infancy', *British Journal of Nutrition*, 62, pp. 621–9.

Dewey, K.G., Heinig, M.J., Nommsen, L.A. and Lonnerdale, B. (1991), 'Maternal versus infant factors related to breast milk intake and residual milk volume: the DARLING study', *Pediatrics*, 87, pp. 829–37.

Dewey, K.G. and Lonnerdal, B. (1986), 'Infant self-regulation of breast milk intake', *Acta Paediatrica Scandinavica*, 75, pp. 893–8.

Drewett, R.F. (1978), 'The development of motivational systems', *Progress in Brain Research*, 48, pp. 407–17.

Drewett, R.F. and Woolridge, M. (1981) 'Milk taken by human babies from the first and second breast', *Physiology and Behaviour*, 26, pp. 327–9.

Drewett, R.F., Woolridge, M.W., Greasley, V., McLead, C.N., Hewison, J., Williams, A.F. and Baum, J.D. (1984), 'Evaluating breast-milk intake by test weighing: a portable electronic balance suitable for community and field studies', *Early Human Development*, 10, pp. 123–6.

Dunn, P.M. and Pollnitz, R. (1975), 'Subsidising national dried milk', *Lancet*, 1, p. 269.

Eaton-Evans, J. and Dugdale, A.E. (1988), 'Sleep patterns of infants in the first year of life', *Archives of Disease in Childhood*, 63, pp. 647–9.

Elias, M.F., Nicolson, N.A., Bora, C. and Johnston, J. (1986), 'Sleep/wake patterns of breast-fed infants in the first 2 years of life', *Pediatrics*, 77, pp. 322–9.

Ernst, J.A., Rickard, K.A., Neal, P.R., Yu, P-L., Oei, T.O. and Lemons, J.A. (1989), 'Lack of improved growth outcome related to nonnutritive sucking in very low birth weight premature infants fed a controlled nutrient intake: a randomized prospective study', *Journal of Pediatrics*, 83, pp. 706–16.

Fagioli, I., Bes, F. and Salzarulo, P. (1988), '24-hour behavioural state distribution in continuously fed infants', *Early Human Development*, 18, pp. 151–6.

FAO/WHO/UNO (1985), 'Energy and protein requirements', Technical Report Series, No. 724 (Geneva: FAO/WHO/UNO).

Field, T., Ignatoff, E., Stringer, S., Brennan, J., Greenberg, R., Widmayer, S. and Anderson, G.C. (1982), 'Nonnutritive sucking during tube feedings: effects on preterm neonates in an intensive care unit', *Pediatrics*, 70, pp. 381–4.

Fomon, S.J., Filer, L.J., Thomas, L.N., Anderson, T.A. and Nelson, S.E. (1975), 'Influence of formula concentration on caloric intake and growth of normal infants', *Acta Paediatrica Scandinavica*, 64, pp. 172–81.

Fomon, S.J., Filer, L.J., Thomas, L.N., Rogers, R.R. and Proksch, A.M. (1969), 'Relationship between formula concentration and rate of growth of normal infants', *Journal of Nutrition*, 98, pp. 241–54.

Fomon, S.J., Haschke, F., Ziegler, E.E. and Nelson, S.E. (1988), 'Body composition of reference children from birth to age 10 years', *American Journal of Clinical Nutrition*, 35, pp. 1169–75.

Fomon, S.J., Thomas, L.N., Filer, L.J., Anderson, T.A. and Nelson, S.E. (1976), 'Influence of fat and carbohydrate content of diet on food intake and growth of male infants', *Acta Paediatrica Scandinavica*, 65, pp. 136–44.

Gilmore, H.E. and Rowland, T.W. (1978), 'Critical malnutrition in breast-fed infants', *American Journal of Diseases of Children*, 132, pp. 885–7.

Hunt, J.N. (1980), 'A possible relation between the regulation of gastric emptying and food intake', *American Journal of Physiology*, 2, pp. G1–4.

Hunt, J.N. and Stubbs, D.F. (1975), 'The volume and energy content of meals as determinants of gastric emptying', *Journal of Physiology*, 245, pp. 209–25.

Hytten, F.E. (1954), 'Clinical and chemical studies in human lactation VI. The functional capacity of the breast', *British Medical Journal*, 1, pp. 912–15.

Hytten, F.E., Yorston, J.C. and Thomson, A.M. (1958), 'Difficulties associated with breast-feeding: a study of 106 primiparas', *British Medical Journal*, 1, pp. 310–15.

Janovsky, M., Martinek, J. and Stanincova, V. (1967), 'The distribution of sodium, chloride and fluid in the body of the young infants with increased intake of NaCl', *Biologia Neonatorium*, 11, pp. 261–72.

Keesey, R.E. and Powley, T.L. (1986), 'The regulation of body weight', *Annual Review of Psychology*, 37, pp. 109–33.

Lawrence, M., Lawrence, F., Durnin, J.V.G.A. and Whitehead, R.G. (1991), 'A comparison of physical activity in Gambian and UK children aged 6–18 months', *European Journal of Clinical Nutrition*, 45, pp. 243–52.

Lothe, L., Ivarsson, S-.A., Erman, R. and Lindberg, T. (1990), 'Motilin and infantile colic', *Acta Paediatrica Scandinavica*, 79, pp. 410–16.

Lucas, A., Bishop, N.J., King, F. and Cole, T.J. (1992), 'Randomised trial of nutrition for preterm infants after discharge', *Archives of Disease in Childhood*, **67**, pp. 324–7.

Macknin, M.L., Medendorp, S.V. and Maier, M.C. (1989), 'Infant sleep and bedtime cereal', *American Journal of Diseases of Children*, **143**, pp. 1066–8.

Martines, J.C., Rea, M. and de Zoysa, I. (1992), 'Breast feeding in the first six months: no need for extra fluids', *British Medical Journal*, **304**, pp. 1068–9.

Matheny, R.J., Birch, L.L. and Picciano, M.F. (1990), 'Control of milk intake by human-milk-fed infants: relationships between feeding size and interval', *Developmental Psychobiology*, **23**, pp. 511–18.

Measel, C.P. and Anderson, G.C. (1979), 'Nonnutritive sucking during tube feedings: effect on clinical course in premature infants', *Journal of the Nurses Association of the American College of Obstetricians and Gynecologists*, **8**, pp. 265–72.

Miller, J.J., McVeagh, P., Fleet, G.H., Petocz, P. and Brand, J.C. (1989), 'Breath hydrogen secretion in infants with colic', *Archives of Disease in Childhood*, **64**, pp. 725–9.

Morley, D. and Woodland, M. (1979) *See How They Grow* (London: Macmillan).

Neifert, M.R., Seacat, J.M. and Jobe, W.E. (1985), 'Lactation failure due to insufficient glandular development of the breast', *Pediatrics*, **76**, pp. 823–8.

Ostrander, C.R., Cohen, R.S., Hopper, A.O., Shahin, S.M., Kerner, J.A., Johnson, J.D. and Stevenson, D.K. (1983), 'Breath hydrogen analysis: a review of the methodologies and clinical applications', *Journal of Pediatric Gastroenterology and Nutrition*, **2**, pp. 525–33.

Ounsted, M. and Sleigh, G. (1975), 'The infant's self-regulation of food intake and weight gain', *Lancet*, **1**, pp. 1393–7.

Pollitt, E., Gilmore, M. and Valcarel, M. (1978), 'Early mother–infant interaction and somatic growth', *Early Human Development*, **1**, pp. 325–36.

Prechtl, H.F.R. (1958), 'The directed head turning response and allied movements of the human baby', *Behaviour*, **13**, pp. 212–42.

Prentice, A.M., Lucas, A., Vasquez-Velasquez, L., Davies, P.S.W. and Whitehead, R.G. (1988), 'Are current dietary guidelines for young children a prescription for overfeeding?', *Lancet*, **11**, pp. 1066–9.

Roberts, D.F. (1981), 'Genetics of growth', in J.M. Tanner (ed.), *Control of Growth* (London: Churchill Livingstone).

Roberts, S.B., Savage, J., Coward, W.A., Chew, B. and Lucas, A. (1988), 'Energy expenditure and intake in infants born to lean and overweight mothers', *New England Journal of Medicine*, **318**, pp. 461–6.

St. James-Roberts, I. (1989), 'Persistent crying in infancy', *Journal of Child Psychology and Psychiatry*, **30**, pp. 189–95.

Salzarulo, P., Fagioli, I. and Ricour, C. (1980), 'Long term continuously fed infants do not develop heart rate circadian rhythm', *Early Human Development*, **12**, pp. 285–9.

Smith, D.W., Truog, W., Rogers, J.E., Greitzer, L.J., Skinner, A.L., McCann, J.J. and Harvey, M.A.S. (1976), 'Shifting linear growth during infancy: illustration of genetic factors in growth from fetal life through infancy', *Journal of Pediatrics*, **89**, pp. 225–30.

Taitz, L.S. and Byers, H.D. (1972), 'High calorie/osmolar feeding and hypertonic dehydration', *Archives of Disease in Childhood*, **47**, pp. 257–60.

Tanner, J.M. (1981), 'Catch-up growth in man', in J.M. Tanner (ed.), *Control of Growth* (London: Churchill Livingstone).

Tanner, J.M. (1986), 'Growth as a target-seeking function. Catch-up and catch-down growth in man', in F. Falkner and J.M. Tanner (eds), *Human Growth, vol. 1 Developmental Biology, Prenatal Growth*, pp. 167–79.

Tyson, J., Burchfield, J., Sentance, F., Mize, C., Uauy, R. and Eastburn, J. (1992), 'Adaptation of feeding to a low fat yield in breast milk', *Pediatrics*, **89**, pp. 215–20.

Vasquez-Velasquez, L. (1988), 'Energy expenditure and physical activity of malnourished Gambian infants', *Proceedings of the Nutrition Society*, **47**, pp. 233–9.

Wailoo, M.P., Peterson, S.A. and Whittaker, H. (1990), 'Disturbed nights in 3–4 month old infants – the effects of feeding and thermal environment', *Archives of Disease in Childhood*, **65**, pp. 499–501.

Waterlow, J.C. and Thomson, A.M. (1979), 'Observations on the adequacy of breast-feeding', *Lancet*, **2**, pp. 238–41.

Whitehead, R.G., Paul, A.A. and Cole, T.J. (1982), 'How much breast milk do babies need?', *Acta Paediatrica Scandinavica*, Supplement, **291**, pp. 43–50.

Wolff, P.H. (1968), 'The serial organization of sucking in the young infant', *Pediatrics*, **42**, pp. 943–56.

Woolridge, M. and Drewett, R.F. (1986), 'Sucking rates of human babies on the breast; a study using direct observation and intraoral pressure measurements', *Journal of Reproductive and Infant Psychology*, **4**, pp. 69–75.

World Health Organization (1983), *Measuring Change in Nutritional Status* (Geneva: W.H.O.).

Wright, P., Fawcett, J.N. and Crow, R.A. (1980), 'The development of differences in the feeding behaviour of bottle and breast-fed human infants from birth to two months', *Behavioural Processes*, **5**, pp. 1–20.

Wright, P., MacLeod, H.A. and Cooper, M.J. (1983), 'Waking at night: the effect of early feeding experience', *Child: Care, Health and Development*, **9**, pp. 309–19.

Yorston, J.C. and Hytten, F.E. (1957), 'Rapid gastric emptying time as a cause of crying in breast-fed babies', *Proceedings of the Nutrition Society*, **16**, p. vi.

Ziegler, E.E. and Fomon, S.J. (1971), 'Fluid intake, renal solute load and water balance in infancy', *Journal of Pediatrics*, **78**, pp. 561–8.

Chapter 5

Mothers' ideas about feeding in early infancy

Peter Wright, *University of Edinburgh*

The extent to which the state of hunger is uniquely characterised by particular behaviours in the young infant, and whether these behaviours are correctly interpreted and acted on by the mother, is a question which has been of some interest to psychologists (Wright, 1987a). Feeding can be a source of great anxiety to many mothers. Several studies have commented on the very high incidence of consultations by mothers with a physician in the first three months of life, in which the chief concern of the mother has been feeding difficulties. Some estimates are that as many as 30 per cent of mothers will present such problems either to a health visitor or a GP (Sumner and Fritsch, 1977; Forsyth *et al.*, 1985; Pridham, 1987). Mothers who are particularly anxious or depressed, as measured by a state and trait anxiety inventory, may doubt their own competence in looking after their babies and may tend to believe that their own breast milk is inadequate (Hellin and Waller, 1992). Anxious mothers perceived their babies as fussy, hungry and demanding, and in particular expressed concern about milk regurgitation at the end of feeds.

A special concern of health professionals is the continuing need to encourage mothers to take up and persist with breast-feeding their infant until at least three months of age. Although there has recently been considerable improvement in the proportion of women who commence breast-feeding in hospital (Martin and Monk, 1982), survey after survey reports a dramatic drop in this proportion within a few weeks of leaving hospital. There is universal encouragement of breast-feeding on the hospital wards, and although large numbers of mothers may breast-feed when in hospital, one third of those mothers will have given up by six weeks after delivery (Martin and White, 1988; DHSS, 1989).

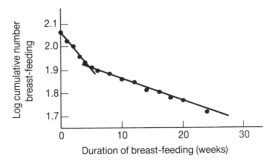

Figure 5.1 Log survivorship plot of breast-feeding duration.

The results of a recent Edinburgh survey of breast-feeding duration (Wright, 1990) are shown in Fig. 5.1, as a survivorship analysis, a technique which is widely used in medical research. In this particular instance a logarithmic scale has been used to make the picture easier to interpret.

The break in the curve at around six weeks of age suggests there are two different populations, and the slope of the line shows that the probability that mothers will terminate breast-feeding is high in the first six weeks. At around the six-week point, however, there is an abrupt change in the slope and the mothers who 'survive' into the period beyond six weeks are much less likely to give up. Therefore six weeks may be a critical point or hurdle, which if surmounted means that a mother is likely to continue to breast-feed for the recommended period of four to six months. The author has argued elsewhere (Wright, 1987b) that mothers need to be more aware of some of the behaviours associated with breast-feeding at this critical time, such as a changed pattern in feeds, and in particular increased frequency of feeds towards the end of the afternoon and early evening. From birth to around four weeks of age, the amount of breast milk taken at each feed is very similar. This changes by eight weeks to a pronounced diurnal pattern of feeding, with large feeds taken at the beginning of the day and feeds becoming progressively smaller throughout the day (Wright *et al.*, 1980; Wright, 1986, 1987c).

Mothers' beliefs about feeding

There are initial differences between bottle- and breast-feeding mothers which, in the latter case, predispose them to elect to breast-feed in the first place, and which in themselves may account for some differences in the behaviour of breast- and bottle-fed infants (Richards and Bernal, 1971; Switzky *et al.*, 1979).

The two groups differ in their expectations, in the aspects of feeding they view as important, and especially in their concern regarding the 'psychological environment'. Breast-feeding mothers express more concern that feeding should be an enjoyable experience in a relaxed atmosphere for both the mother and the infant (Crow, 1977; Berg-Cross and McGeehan, 1979; Kearney *et al.*, 1990). Why this difference? Is it because in encouraging mothers to breast-feed, midwives and health visitors stress these processes? Or is it something that mothers have read about in the lay literature? The finding may have important implications for practice since, if this is an expectation of how breast-feeding should be experienced, does it in fact reflect reality? On numerous occasions we have heard mothers who were breast-feeding complain that it was a pity no-one had warned them that they might feel tired or even uncomfortable when feeding. It is therefore possible that failure to teach such expectations could influence a mother's relationship with her baby and jeopardise the successful outcome of breast-feeding.

How do unsuccessful and successful breast-feeding groups differ? We have not found any differences in the reasons for wanting to breast-feed in the first place, with both groups being equally positive about the perceived benefits of breast-feeding (Wright, 1990). When the reasons for terminating breast-feeding were examined, the majority of our mothers, apart from a few who considered six weeks to be 'successful' and had never intended to feed any longer than this, produced the usual wide range of reasons, in which the claim to have insufficient milk was by far the most common. Because so many studies have the same finding (Sacks *et al.*, 1976; Martin and Monk, 1982; Holt and Wolkind, 1983) there is a very real possibility that the belief becomes common knowledge in the community and that, despite their knowledge of the physiology of lactation, many nurses may have the sneaking suspicion that it is a belief based on fact.

Beliefs are powerful determinants of behaviour. This applies as much to regulation of our own food intake as it does to a mother's view of feeding her own infant. Sometimes these beliefs may conform with actual behaviour, but on other occasions can be at variance with this (Rajan, 1986). As an illustration, some newly breast-feeding mothers find advice to allow the infant to suckle frequently very difficult to follow, for example because they may erroneously believe that if they delay feeding more milk will have accumulated in the breast.

Feeding during the first weeks of life is a very different experience for both infant and mother than it is once lactation is firmly established, and it is important for the nursing mother to realise that the behaviour of her infant may differ in characteristic ways from that of a bottle-fed infant of the same age. Mothers inevitably make such comparisons and will continue to do so as they visit postnatal clinics and discuss their experiences with their contemporaries. Some of these differences will be discussed later in this chapter, but suffice to say here that, in the first week of life, breast-fed infants appear more hungry than those bottle fed (Richards and Bernal, 1971), and in the first few days the 24-hour intake of bottle-fed infants is constant, whereas the breast-fed infant experiences a gradual daily increase in intake. Bottle-fed infants consume more milk on the third day of life than do breast-fed babies

Table 5.1 Do babies sleep longer following a large meal?

Age of baby	Breast		Bottle	
	Yes	No	Yes	No
1–2 weeks	17	4	24	2
2–4 months	14	8	20	0

and in a biological sense can be said to have consumed too much (Crow and Wright, 1976). Three- and four-day-old infants do not sleep longer after they have a large feed, and mothers cannot therefore guarantee a peaceful night by giving the baby an extra ounce of milk. However, mothers of both breast- and bottle-fed infants believe that babies will sleep longer after a large meal, a significant mismatch between infant behaviour and mothers' beliefs (see Table 5.1).

Feeding during infancy has been held to be a period free from the influence of cognitive, social and cultural factors (Garrow, 1978). Indeed, the Royal College Report on Obesity explicitly stated that one way of assessing the physiological control of food intake in man, while limiting the effects of social pressures, is to monitor the intake of the neonate and the growing child (Royal College of Physicians, 1983). Unfortunately this view of infant feeding behaviour operating within a cultural vacuum is misplaced. Infant feeding cannot be dissociated from mother–infant interaction during feeding, and mothers invariably have firm beliefs about infant feeding practice.

In the Third World, continuous physical contact between mother and infant is usual, making the breast routinely available in response to subtle signals from the child (Vis and Hennart, 1978). In a survey of infant care practices in hunter–gatherer and other non-industrialised societies, Lozoff and Brittenham (1979) found similar behaviours encouraging close contact in all of the former and over 50 per cent of the latter. Modernisation brings with it structural changes in the environment, such as separate sleeping quarters and technological devices in which to 'cache' an infant. Quandt (1986) in a North American study reported an association between lower breast-feeding frequency in houses with many rooms compared to greater feeding frequency in compact dwellings. Mothers reported that waking infants often spent a considerable time making low noises with stretching, grunting and sucking before a full cry. Consistently responding before the full cry is more possible in the compact than in the dispersed dwellings and results in reduced between-feeding intervals and increased feeding frequency.

Feeding a a developing skill

As feeding infants is an acquired skill, mothers must have some means of selecting appropriate patterns of behaviour from a repertoire of possible courses of action. Crow (1977) suggested that a useful schema for viewing infant feeding is to break down the practice into the categories of plans, actions, and observed behaviour of the infant (see Fig. 5.2).

The plan is likely to incorporate ideas about the type of food babies should have, how much food they should take, and how frequently they should be fed. Together these ideas reflect the mother's concept of infant feeding which is itself derived from such sources as past experience, baby books and magazines, cultural practices and medical advice, etc. (Crow and Wright, 1976). The plan becomes operational through the mother's actions, i.e. those behaviours used to carry out the mother's intentions. For example, she may pick up the baby immediately he/she begins to cry, or feed with a spoon for the first time, or wind the baby. But the particular form these actions will take depends not only upon the mother's concept of feeding, but also on the baby's behaviour, and so a third category within this framework is the baby's observed behaviour.

Feedback from the infant functions at two levels. Feedback A provides the necessary information needed for actions to be successfully performed, e.g. responding if the baby's nose is obstructed by the breast when feeding. Feedback B involves evaluating the baby's state. As a result of this assessment, decisions are made about whether to continue with the same course of action, to try something else, or to stop. For example, if the baby falls asleep but there is still a considerable amount of milk left in the bottle, a decision has to be made about whether the feed should be terminated or the baby woken up to take more. Furthermore, for this form of feedback, not only will current information be used, but a comparison will also be made to see whether the results of the action match up to the expected outcome. A discrepancy with the expected outcome leads to a change in the course of action, whilst a match will ensure either a continuation of what is being done, or that the practice will be terminated. In other words, whilst feedback A is used to maintain a particular action, feedback B is used to make decisions about any changes that are required.

Satter (1990) and Pridham (1990) provide an interesting discussion of the developmental principles guiding feeding in the first year of life; in this they describe the initial requirement to achieve homeostasis, or regulation of state.

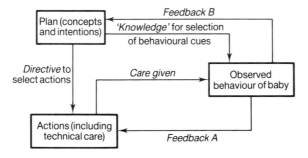

Figure 5.2 Schematic representation of infant feeding.

The process of feeding enables behaviour in the newborn to become more organised, the mother calms and organises the infant by following feeding cues, and works to keep the infant in a quiet alert state. One can view such interactions as being in the zone of proximal development, a phase prior to independent performance, in which a child who has some skills needed for a task can accomplish the task with the assistance of a more capable person (Wertsch, 1984). A mother may assess the infant's cues as to getting the feeding started, pacing and terminating the feeding. Tacitly operating in the zone of proximal development, mothers may arrange and support the feeding interaction such that infants can manage components of the feeding on their own terms (Pridham *et al.*, 1989).

Changes in the sucking patterns of infants have potential signal value as expressions of both hunger and satiety. Peiper (1961) considered satiety as a negation of those aspects concerned with hunger, an absence of the rooting reflex and a gradual increase in the pause length between sucks. Associated with this reduction in sucking is a motor restlessness when the infant may release the nipple or push it out with the tongue. This particular expression of satiety he felt was only suited to breast-fed babies. While satiety is a response both to food intake and to fatigue, Peiper argued the latter was the more efficient mechanism. When no effort is required, only very large intakes will induce satiety and, because bottle-feeding is less effortful, Peiper argued that bottle-fed babies are in greater danger of overfeeding.

Dubignon and Campbell (1969) showed that fatigue and satiation do have separate effects within the first week of life in bottle-fed infants, but not on sucking *per se*. Babies who have had enough or who are tired will reduce the amount of time they spend sucking, but will not alter the rate at which they suck. Dubignon and Campbell attributed this decrease in time spent sucking to both satiation and fatigue, as recovery, following stops for winding, occurred throughout the feed, not just at the start. Satiation is independently expressed by refusal of the bottle. Sucking is therefore not the most reliable index of satiety because it can be confused with fatigue and level of arousal.

Responding to infant signals in breast- and bottle-feeding

The single most important variable likely to influence the development of feeding behaviour is initial choice of feeding method. In terms of the infant-feeding schema outlined above, there are immediate differences in the nature of the feedback available to the mother, with the most salient being awareness of amount consumed, knowledge of which is only indirectly available to the breast-feeding mother. The medical and paediatric literature emphasise the compositional differences between breast milk and artificial formula, with professional advice at pains to ensure that mothers correctly make up formula to the appropriate dilution.

Choice of feeding method results in differences in the pacing of feeds which seem related to the establishment of control over actions by the infant. Wright *et al.* (1980) analysed the interruptions within filmed feeds caused by the removal of the bottle or breast for a variety of reasons such as choking, winding, possetting of milk, changing breast, etc. Each interruption was scored in terms of it being either mother or baby determined, at one week, one month and two months. Whereas in bottle-fed babies the interruptions were almost entirely under the control of the mother, in contrast there was a predominantly baby-determined pattern for the breast feeds. These results agree with earlier observations of Dunn (1975) on one-week-old infants. Although inexperience on the part of the mother could in part account for such interruptions at one week, this is unlikely to be the case with older infants, suggesting a lack of reciprocity. In most reports, nursing dyads display more reciprocity in the context of feeding than do their bottle-fed counterparts (Dunn and Richards, 1977; Crow *et al.*, 1981; Walton and Vallelunga, 1989).

At this gross level of analysis, it is clear that the role of the baby in indicating satiety by terminating feeds at an early point in the satiety sequence is minimised in the case of the bottle-fed baby. All such decision making remains the prerogative of the mother, and there is no indication of any developmental change across the first two months of life. In the case of the breast-fed baby there seems a far greater degree of flexibility. When mothers were asked about the criteria used to decide when their baby had had enough milk (Wright, 1990), falling asleep was recognised as a satiety cue more commonly by breast-feeding mothers, with more bottle-feeding mothers terminating feeds only when the baby spits out the teat. These answers become interesting when considered in relation to direct observations of infant feeding behaviour. There seem to be several stages in the process of terminating a feed – the baby slows down its sucking rate, becomes drowsy and, if mother still continues the feed, will refuse to open its mouth or will spit out the teat if it is forced into the mouth. In terms of this progression it would appear that some bottle-feeding mothers are more likely to override the early signals of satiety and are thus in greater danger of overfeeding their baby. Interpreted in these terms, this finding would be an example of an environmental factor that could contribute to the development of rapid weight gain and obesity (Wright, 1981).

Mothers' recognition of hunger during infancy

Are mothers themselves aware of any differences in their baby's level of hunger across the day? When mothers attending routine baby clinics are asked this and other questions relating to awareness of their own milk supply and their baby's hunger signals, breast-feeding mothers are far more likely to report hunger variation than are bottle-feeding mothers (Wright, 1988). Whereas 82 per cent of mothers breast-feeding eight-week-old infants commonly experience a time of day when they report increased hunger in their infants, only 57 per cent of bottle-feeding mother report any such variation (see Fig. 5.3). Breast-feeding mothers also report hunger variation significantly more often in female infants, but no such sex difference is apparent in the bottle-feeding mothers (see Table 5.2).

Table 5.2 Is there variation in hunger across the day?

Sex	Breast only[1]		Bottle only[2]	
	Yes	No	Yes	No
Male	36	15	16	14
Female	42	2	27	18

1. $X^2 = 8.32$, df 1, $p < 0.01$.
2. $X^2 = 0.11$, df 1, NS.

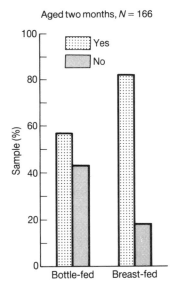

Figure 5.3 Presence of hunger variation in breast- and bottle-fed infants.

When mothers are asked why they report variations in hunger across the day, they put forward a wide range of behaviours and reasons which can be classified into five categories (Wright, 1987c).

1. *Avidity measures.* Comments concerning the intensity of the sucking or the speed or length of sucking: 'desperate, sucks everything'; 'sucks rapidly'; 'sucks slowly and rhythmically'.

2. *Distractability.* The baby is said to be more hungry because it is less distractable and more singleminded about the feed: 'gets on with it'; 'sustained concentration'; 'no rests for looking about'.
3. *Cries and screams.* 'screams until fed'.
4. *Very frequent feeding.* The baby demands feeds more frequently: 'fed in under three hours'; 'wants lots of little feeds'; 'has to be fed very often'.
5. *Maternal inference.* The mother makes an inference to support her claim for increased hunger at this stage of the day: 'has gone all night without food, and so must be more hungry'.

Of those bottle-feeding mothers who did report awareness of hunger variation (see Fig. 5.4), vigour of sucking was by far the most common reason offered. Increased frequency of feeding or demands for feeds was the most common reason offered by the breast-feeding mothers. A further marked contrast between the two feeding techniques at this age is the time of day when mothers consider their baby to be most hungry (see Fig. 5.5.).

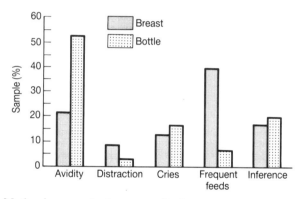

Figure 5.4 Mothers' reasons for hunger attribution.

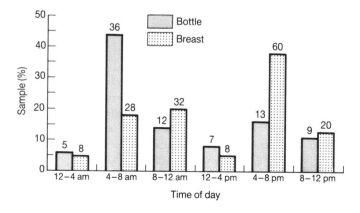

Figure 5.5 Time of day when mother believes infant is most hungry.

Bottle-feeding mothers cite feeds at the beginning of the day, often after the overnight fast, as the time when their baby is most hungry, whereas the breast-feeding mothers highlight late afternoon as the most hungry time.

Wright (1987a) described the two-month-old breast-fed infant as essentially responding to a defecit signal and compensating for the long night interval without milk. In a reanalysis of existing data, Matheny *et al.* (1990) found preprandial correlations between meal size and interval since the last feed in breast-fed infants, which they likewise describe as a reactive-type feeding pattern. Wright (1981) found that in older breast-fed infants, aged between four and six months, there is no longer a pattern of largest feed in the morning and a progressive decrease throughout the day. The largest feed now occurs at the end of the day. This change may result from the infant actively learning to anticipate periods of absence of food by taking larger meals ahead of the long night-time fast. It was suggested that this move from an early more primitive form of defecit responding in the infant shifts with age to an anticipatory mode in the older infant. Similar changes in meal size have been reported in a bottle-fed infant (Wright, 1987a). As there was neither restriction in the availability of milk or any variation in milk composition in the case of the bottle-fed infant, this suggests that such cues are an unlikely explanation for age changes seen in the breast-feeding pattern, and provide support for the idea of active learning as an explanation.

Gender differences in feeding

At eight weeks of age there is a significantly greater frequency of feeding male infants in the early hours of the morning, and of girls being fed more frequently towards the end of the day. This finding comes from studies in which mothers kept careful records of all breast-feeds over a four-day period. In Fig. 5.6 these are plotted as the mean frequency of feeds which were initiated within successive four-hour periods across the day, commencing at midnight.

The observation of an increased frequency of feeding in two-month-old breast-fed male infants by comparison with females during the antisocial early morning hours is also confirmed in reanalysis of data provided by the authors of a study on night waking and the thermal environment in three- to four-month-old infants (Wailoo *et al.*, 1990). Parents completed a prospective diary of a night's sleep at home for 87 infants with an average age of 14.9 weeks, and thermistor probes were affixed to record body temperature continuously at four sites in addition to ambient temperature. In view of the commitment involved, it is likely that the parents were particularly careful in recording accurately all instances of waking and feeding at the time of occurrence.

Wailoo *et al.* confirm that breast-fed infants were more likely to disturb

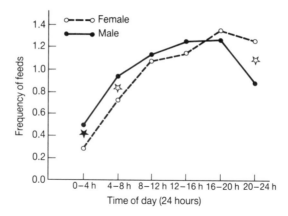

Figure 5.6 Mean frequency of feeds in each consecutive four-hour period plotted across a 24-hour day. Black star, $p < 0.05$; white star, $p < 0.01$.

their parents in the early hours of the morning ($X^2 = 5.9$, $3df$, $p < 0.01$). What is particularly interesting in their data is, first, the lack of any difference in the frequency of wakings between midnight and 6 am as a function of infant gender (39 male, 43 recorded wakings; 46 female, 48 recorded wakings). However, whereas this waking led to male infants feeding on 68 per cent of occasions, females were fed on only 45 per cent of occasions (see Table 5.3(a)). As most of the babies in the sample were still being breast-fed at the time of measurement, the same analysis can be made on those entirely bottle-feeding (see Table 5.3(b)). Again, male infants were significantly more likely to be fed than female.

Table 5.3 (a) Waking at night between 12 and 6 am (from Wailoo *et al.*, 1990).

	Male	Female
Fed	24	16
Not fed	15	30

$X^2 = 5.04$, df 1, $p < 0.02$.

(b) Bottle-fed infants only.

	Male	Female
Fed	18	10
Not fed	11	27

$X^2 = 6.8$, df 1, $p < 0.01$.

The Tog values of clothing worn before putting the babies down for the night were also assessed, and babies who disturbed their parents more than once were significantly more heavily wrapped than those who slept through or woke only once. Subsequent to this present reanalysis of the sex differences in feeding in this study, a significant difference in the Tog value of the clothing of males and females was detected (male $13.1 + 0.6$; female $15.1 + 0.8$, $p < 0.01$, Student's t test. Petersen, personal communication).

In this study, therefore, with a mixed population of ages and feeding method, the same finding of increased frequency of feeding male infants in the early hours of the morning is reported. As this was equally true of those who were formula fed, it would seem that the greater leniency towards male infants' feeding demands is not only present in mothers breast-feeding their infants but in those bottle-feeding as well.

There are no reported sex differences in the incidence of breast-feeding amongst mothers of term infants and surprisingly gender was not a variable considered in any of the OPCS surveys within the United Kingdom (Martin and Monk, 1982; Martin and White, 1988). However, Lucas et al. (1988) found that mothers were significantly more likely to provide breast-milk for boys. Sumner and Fritsch (1977) monitored telephone requests for medical information by new parents in the immediate postnatal period and noted there were twice as many requests for information about the breast-feeding of boys than girls. A similar sex imbalance was reported by Adebonojo (1972) with respect to reports for information on bottle-feeding. Although it might be argued that some parents would be aware of the poorer clinical outcome for premature male infants, the notion of increased male vulnerability is not widely known, and these studies may either reflect greater difficulty in dealing with boys in the immediate postnatal period or, alternatively, that mothers put greater investment into the care of male than female infants.

Long-term associations with early feeding practice

There has already been some mention in this chapter of the possible connection between early feeding experience and later developmental outcome. Three issues will be briefly touched on here: the first concerns subsequent physical growth, the second the issue of sleeping through the night, and the third recent claims with respect to intellectual development.

Growth

Although lacking conclusive evidence, there is a widespread belief amongst clinicians that breast-feeding minimises the risk of rapid weight gain and subsequent obesity because the control of milk intake rests with the baby rather than with the mother, and that in addition the mother is ignorant as to the exact amount of milk consumed (Kramer, 1981). The bottle-feeding mother always has immediate feedback as to how much milk has been taken from the bottle. In a series of experiments, Fomon and colleagues asked what would happen if the mother was unaware as to the true nature of the formula and did not have explicit instructions about how much to offer at each feed (Fomon *et al.*, 1969, 1975). Would bottle-feeding mothers under these circumstances allow their infants to determine intake, and would the babies compensate for changes in the strength of the feed? In discussing these results, Fomon (1980) stated, 'the babies found out what was going wrong, and they fixed it', and they have been taken to imply that the infant has the capacity to regulate its intake after about six weeks of age (Taitz, 1983; Pollitt *et al.*, 1981; Birch, 1987). If the regulation revealed in Fomon *et al.*'s experiments is by the infant rather than the mother, we still do not have any information on how this has been achieved. For example, are the infants adjusting their intake by varying the number of meals each day, or by the amount taken at each meal? And, if the latter, are the mothers perhaps attending to cues earlier in the satiety sequence because of their lack of guidance on appropriate intake each day, rather than feeding to the point of final satiety indicated by spitting out the teat?

Such questions are important because, whereas the size of feeds does not vary across the day in bottle-fed infants (Wright *et al.*, 1980), for breast-feeding infants pronounced diurnal patterns of meal size appear by approximately eight weeks of age (Wright *et al.*, 1980; Pao *et al.*, 1980; Butte *et al.*, 1985). The largest meals occur in the early morning, and the smallest meals at the end of the day. This pattern is in marked contrast to that of approximately equal-sized meals found at four weeks of age, with the changes corresponding to the critical six-week period referred to at the start of this chapter, a point at which many mothers cease to breast-feed. As Drewett points out (see Chapter 4), this does not necessarily reflect decreased hunger on the part of the infant across the day, as the changed milk intakes may be due either to variation in appetite or to the mother's milk-producing capacity.

Sleeping

From both prospective (Wright, 1981) and retrospective (Wright *et al.*, 1983) studies, there is clear evidence that mothers who elect to bottle-feed their infants from birth will find that the feeds which occur in the early hours of the morning are dropped at a significantly earlier age. It is always difficult to support the contention that differences observed between feeding type classification groups (breast and bottle) are a result of early feeding experience *per se*, rather than being produced by a secondary association with social class. These authors showed that, although their sample had the usual statistical relationship between social class and feeding method, there was no independent effect of social class on night waking. Wright *et al.* (1983) focused on what they described as 'asocial' hours of the night (between midnight and six am), and they found that such feeds stop on average in bottle-fed infants at around ten weeks of age and in breast-fed infants at sixteen weeks. This difference is especially significant for the advice on introduction of solids which is offered to mothers.

Generally, physicians and health professionals advise delaying the intro-duction of solids until the infant is at least 3–4 months old. Despite this advice, bottle-feeding mothers consistently introduce solids earlier than do breast-feeding mothers. A very common reason offered by such mothers is that of resumed night waking (Wright *et al.*, 1983). As more bottle-fed infants develop a pattern of sleeping through the night by the age of three months, disruption of this pattern by resumed night waking will be viewed by the mother with dismay and interpreted, rightly or wrongly, as the infant needing food other than milk. It is therefore hardly surprising that bottle-feeding mothers disregard the professional advice offered in the face of a far more persuasive argument, namely the changed behaviour of their infant. Because such a pattern of consistent sleeping is not so likely to be present in the breast-fed infant at this age, the advice to delay the introduction of solids is therefore entirely compatible with the infant's behaviour.

When mothers of nursery school children were questioned about their child's current feeding and sleeping habits, Wright *et al.* (1983) found that those children who continued to wake at night were likely to be those who had been previously breast-fed, and this was not attributable to social class influences. The authors' explanation of why night waking should persist in a previously breast-fed population is analogous to that already proposed to account for the earlier introduction of solids by the bottle-feeding mothers. In general terms, events which parents deem to be a 'problem' will depend on their past experience of their child's behaviour. If an infant which has previously settled into a pattern of sleeping through the night begins to wake again, then a problem will be perceived (the child is hungry?) and a solution sought in terms of the introduction of solid feeds. If, on the other hand, the child has not settled into a pattern of sleeping through the night, continued disturbed nights will not be a cause of anxiety. Therefore, night waking is more probable in a setting in which the mother is less likely to perceive its occurrence as a problem. On this basis, the bottle-feeding mother is more likely to perceive early episodes of night waking as a situation desirous of a solution, and be more ready and able than the breast-feeding mother to apply any necessary negative reinforcement.

Intellectual development

Interruptions within feeds are one of the best examples of how breast-feeding permits a greater degree of control to become established by the infant rather than by the mother. Lewis and Goldberg (1969) have developed the view that the extent to which the environment is contingent on the actions of the infant will determine the strength of his belief that his actions can affect the environment. The infant with a strong expectation of mastery will expect his interactions with the environment to be rewarding, and will be motivated to achieve control through all the means open to him. Establishment of control over interruptions within feeds may be a prototypical example of such mastery. It is interesting to speculate that the claims for a slight IQ advantage associated with breast-feeding which have been attributed to the composition of breast milk (Rodgers, 1978; Taylor and Wadsworth, 1984; Morley *et al.*, 1988) may in fact be due to these behavioural sequelae making the infant engage differently with the environment. The ability to control actions is considered to be an important ingredient of cognitive development (Piaget, 1950; Bower, 1977; Yarrow and Messer, 1983; Donaldson, 1978) which is not dependent solely upon rewards for progression.

In a recent follow-up study of a large cohort of premature infants, all of which were initially fed different formulae, it was reported that the babies whose mothers supplied their own breast milk had a significantly higher IQ at the age of eight years (Lucas *et al.*, 1992). Because for most of these mothers the breast milk was fed entirely by nasogastric tube, the authors concluded that the composition of breast milk rather than the 'process' of breast-feeding was responsible for the improved IQ. This is undoubtedly an important result and requires further research, but does not exclude the importance of infant mastery outlined above, and does not rule out the obvious competing hypothesis that the IQ advantage of the breast-milk-fed children is attributable to their mothers' high IQs (Wright and Deary, 1992). A similar long-term follow-up of premature infants in Australia found no advantage on psychological test scores for those infants receiving expressed breast-milk, but higher test scores in the children who had received direct breast-feeding (Doyle *et al.*, 1992). This is in agreement with the view put forward above that the act of direct breast-feeding provides benefits for subsequent intellectual development.

Conclusions

In conclusion, there are important differences in the behaviour of infants as a function of feeding method which have implications for professional advice and for the promotion of successful breast-feeding. These include the earlier cessation of night feeds in the bottle-fed infant, the development of pronounced diurnal patterns of breast-feeds by about two months of age, and characteristic differences in the signals which mothers label as indicative of hunger. Surprisingly little accurate knowledge concerning the developmental changes associated with breast-feeding is known to either health professionals or to mothers. This has implications for many practical problems such as sleeping through the night, the introduction of solids, and the reassurance of anxious mothers seeking advice on feeding difficulties. As we improve our understanding of these developmental changes, then so will we be in a better position to forewarn mothers of likely changes in feeding patterns. This will hopefully allow more mothers to successfully breast-feed throughout early infancy, and decrease the large number who discontinue breast-feeding in the belief that they have insufficient milk.

References

Adebonojo, F.O. (1972), 'Artificial versus breastfeeding', *Clinical Pediatrics*, 11, pp. 25–9.

Berg-Cross, L. and McGeehan, D. (1979), 'Experience and personality differences among breast- and bottle-feeding mothers', *Psychology of Women Quarterly*, 3, pp. 344–56.

Birch, L.L. (1987), 'The acquisition of food acceptance patterns in children', in R.A. Boakes, M.J. Burton and D.A. Popplewell (eds), *Eating Habits* (Chichester: John Wiley), pp. 107–30.

Bower, T.G.R. (1977), *A Primer of Infant Development* (San Francisco: Freeman).

Butte, N.F., Wills, C. and Jean, C.A. (1985), 'Feeding patterns of exclusively breast-fed infants during the first four months of life', *Early Human Development*, 12, pp. 291–300.

Crow, R.A. (1977), 'An ethological study of the development of infant feeding', *Journal of Advanced Nursing*, 2, pp. 99–109.

Crow, R.A., Fawcett, J.N. and Wright, P. (1981), 'Maternal behaviour during breast and bottle feeding', *Journal of Behavioural Medicine*, 3, pp. 259–77.

Crow, R.A. and Wright, P. (1976), 'The development of feeding behaviour in early infancy', *Nursing Mirror*, 142, pp. 57–9.

DHSS (1989), *Present-Day Practice in Infant Feeding: Third report*, No. 32 (London: HMSO).

Donaldson, M. (1978), *Children's Minds* (London: Fontana).

Doyle, L.W., Rickards, A.L., Kelly, E.A., Ford, G.W. and Callanan, C. (1992), 'Breastfeeding and intelligence', *Lancet*, 339, pp. 744–5.

Dubignon, J. and Campbell, D. (1969), 'Sucking in the newborn during a feed', *Journal of Experimental Child Psychology*, 6, pp. 154–66.

Dunn, J.B. (1975), 'Consistency and change in styles of mothering', in *Ciba Symposium 33, Parent–Infant Interaction* (Amsterdam: Elsevier), pp. 155–70.

Dunn, J.B. and Richards, M.P. (1977), 'Observations on the developing relationship between mother and baby in the neonatal period', in H.R. Schaffer (ed.), *Studies in Mother–Infant Interaction* (New York: Academic).

Fomon, S.J. (1980), 'Factors influencing food consumption in the human infant', *International Journal of Obesity*, 4, pp. 348–50.

Fomon, S.J., Filer, L.J., Thomas, L.N., Anderson, T.A. and Nelson, S.E. (1975), 'Influence of formula concentration on caloric intake and growth of normal infants', *Acta Paediatrica Scandinavica*, 64, pp. 172–81.

Fomon, S.J., Filer, L.J., Thomas, L.N., Rogers, R.R. and Proksch, A.M. (1969), 'Relationship between formula concentration and rate of growth of normal infants', *Journal of Nutrition*, 98, pp. 241–54.

Forsyth, B.W.C., Leventhal, J.M. and McCarthy, P.L. (1985), 'Mothers' perceptions of problems of feeding and crying behaviors', *American Journal of Diseases in Childhood*, **139**, pp. 269–72.

Garrow, J.S. (1978), 'The regulation of energy expenditure in man', in G. Bray (ed.), *Recent Advances in Obesity Research II* (London: Newman), pp. 200–10.

Hellin, K. and Waller, G. (1992), 'Mothers' mood and infant feeding: prediction of problems and practices', *Journal of Reproductive and Infant Psychology*, **10**, pp. 39–51.

Holt, G.M. and Wolkind, S.N. (1983), 'Early abandonment of breastfeeding: causes and effects', *Child: Care, Health and Development*, **9**, pp. 349–55.

Kearney, M.H., Cronenwett, L.R. and Barrett, J.A. (1990), 'Breast-feeding problems in the first week postpartum', *Nursing Research*, **39**, pp. 90–5.

Kramer, M.S. (1981), 'Do breast-feeding and delayed introduction of solid foods protect against subsequent obesity?', *Journal of Pediatrics*, **98**, pp. 883–7.

Lewis, M. and Goldberg, S. (1969), 'Perceptual–cognitive development in infancy: a generalized expectancy model as a function of the mother–infant interaction', *Merrill-Palmer Quarterly of Behaviour and Development*, **15**, pp. 81–100.

Lozoff, B. and Brittenham, G. (1979). 'Infant care: cache or carry', *Journal of Pediatrics*, **95**, pp. 478–81.

Lucas, A., Cole, T.J., Morley, R., Lucas, P.J., Davis, J.A., Bamford, M.F., Crawle, P., Dossetor, J.F.B., Pearse, R. and Boon, A. (1988), 'Factors associated with maternal choice to provide breast milk for low birthweight infants', *Archives of Disease in Childhood*, **63**, pp. 48–52.

Lucas, A., Morley, R., Cole, T.J., Lister, G. and Leeson-Payne, C. (1992), 'Breast milk and subsequent intelligence quotient in children born before preterm', *Lancet*, **339**, pp. 261–4.

Martin, J. and Monk, J. (1982), *Infant Feeding 1980*, Office of Population Censuses and Surveys, Social Survey Division (London: HMSO).

Martin, J. and White, A. (1988), *Infant Feeding 1985*, Office of Population Censuses and Surveys, Social Survey Division (London: HMSO).

Matheny, R.J., Birch, L.L. and Picciano, M.F. (1990), 'Control of intake by human-milk-fed infants: relationships between feeding size and interval', *Developmental Psychobiology*, **23**, pp. 511–18.

Morley, R., Cole, T.J., Powell, R. and Lucas, A. (1988), 'Mother's choice to provide basic breast milk and developmental outcome', *Archives of Disease in Childhood*, **63**, pp. 1382–5.

Pao, E.M., Himes, J.M. and Roche, A.F. (1980), 'Milk intake and feeding patterns of breast-fed infants', *Journal of the American Dietetic Association*, **77**, pp. 540–5.

Peiper, A. (1961), *Cerebral Functions in Infancy and Childhood* (London: Pitman).

Piaget, J. (1950), *The Psychology of Intelligence* (London: Routledge and Kegan Paul).

Pollitt, E., Consolazio, B. and Goodkin, F. (1981), 'Changes in nutritive sucking during a feed in two day and thirty-two day old infants', *Early Human Development*, **5**, pp. 201–10.

Pridham, K.F. (1987), 'Meaning of infant feeding issues and mothers' use of help', *Journal of Reproductive and Infant Psychology*, **5**, pp. 145–52.

Pridham, K.F. (1990), 'Feeding behaviour of 6- to 12-month old infants: assessment and sources of parental information', *Journal of Pediatrics*, **117**, pp. S174–80.

Pridham, K.F., Knight, C.B. and Stephenson, G.R. (1989), 'Mothers' working models of infant feeding: description and influencing factors', *Journal of Advanced*

Nursing, 14, pp. 1051–61.

Quandt, S.A. (1986), 'Patterns of variation in breast-feeding behaviours', *Social Science and Medicine*, 23, pp. 445–53.

Rajan, L.T. (1986), 'Weaning onto solid foods: mothers' beliefs and practices', *Health Visitor*, 59, pp. 41–4.

Richards, M.P.M. and Bernal, J.F. (1971), 'An observational study of mother–infant interaction', in N. Blurton Jones (ed.), *Ethological Studies of Child Behaviour* (Cambridge: Cambridge University Press).

Rodgers, B. (1978), 'Feeding in infancy and later ability and attainment: a longitudinal study', *Developmental Medicine and Child Neurology*, 20, pp. 421–6.

Royal College of Physicians (1983), 'Obesity: a report of the Royal College of Physicians', *Journal of the Royal College of Physicians of London*, 17, pp. 5–65.

Sacks, S.H., Brada, M., Hill, A.M., Barton, P. and Harland, P.S.E.G. (1976), 'To breast feed or not to breast feed', *Practitioner*, 216, pp. 183–91.

Satter, E. (1990), 'The feeding relationship: problems and interventions', *Journal of Pediatrics*, 117, pp. S181–9.

Sumner, G. and Fritsch, J. (1977), 'Postnatal parental concerns: the first 6 weeks of life', *Journal of Obstetric Gynecological and Neonatal Nursing*, 6, pp. 27–32.

Switzky, L., Vietze, P. and Switzky, H. (1979), 'Attitudinal and demographic predictors of breast-feeding and bottle-feeding behaviour by mothers of six-week-old infants', *Psychological Reports*, 45, pp. 3–14.

Taitz, L.S. (1983), *The Obese Child* (Oxford: Blackwell).

Taylor, B. and Wadsworth, J. (1984), 'Breast-feeding and child development at five years', *Developmental Medicine and Child Neurology*, 26, pp. 73–80.

Vis, H.L. and Hennart, P.L. (1978), 'Decline in breastfeeding: about some of its causes', *Acta paediatrica belgica*, 31, pp. 195–201.

Wailoo, M.P., Petersen, S.A. and Whittaker, H. (1990), 'Disturbed nights in 3–4 month old infants: the effects of feeding and thermal environment', *Archives of Disease in Childhood*, 65, pp. 499–501.

Walton, M.D. and Vallelunga, L.R. (1989), 'The role of breastfeeding in establishing early mother–infant interaction', *Abstracts of the Society for Research in Child Development*, 7, p. 393.

Wertsch, J.V. (1984), 'The zone of proximal development: some conceptual issues', in B. Rogoff and J.V. Wertsch (eds), *Children's Learning in the 'Zone of Proximal Development'*, *New Directions for Child Development*, No. 23 (San Francisco: Jossey-Bass), pp. 7–18.

Wright, P. (1981) 'Development of feeding behaviour in infancy: implications for obesity', *Health Bulletin*, 39, pp. 197–206.

Wright, P. (1986), 'Do mothers know how hungry their babies are?', *Midwifery*, 2, pp. 86–92.

Wright, P. (1987a), 'Hunger, satiety and feeding behaviour in early infancy', in R.A. Boakes, M.J. Burton and D.A. Popplewell (eds), *Eating Habits* (Chichester: John Wiley), pp. 75–105.

Wright, P. (1987b), 'Editorial: breastfeeding behaviour and knowledge', *Journal of Reproductive and Infant Psychology*, 5, pp. 125–6.

Wright, P. (1987c), 'Mother's assessment of hunger in relation to meal size in breastfed infants', *Journal of Reproductive and Infant Psychology*, 5, pp. 173–81.

Wright, P. (1988), 'Learning experiences in feeding behaviour during infancy', *Journal of Psychosomatic Medicine*, 32, pp. 613–19.

Wright, P. (1990), 'Psychological insights into early feeding experience', in A. Faulkner and T. Murphy-Black (eds), *Midwifery: The research route* (London: Scutari), pp. 33–44.

Wright, P. and Deary, I.J. (1992), 'Breastfeeding and intelligence', *Lancet*, **339**, p. 612.

Wright, P., Fawcett, J.N. and Crow, R.A. (1980), 'The development of differences in the feeding behaviour of bottle and breast-fed human infants from birth to two months', *Behavioural Processes*, **5**, pp. 1–20.

Wright, P., Macleod, H.A. and Cooper, M.J. (1983), 'Waking at night: the effect of early feeding experience', *Child: Care, Health and Development*, **9**, pp. 309–19.

Yarrow, L.J. and Messer, D.J. (1983), 'Motivation and cognition in infancy', in M. Lewis (ed.), *Origins of Intelligence*, 2nd edn (New York: Plenum), pp. 951–77.

Chapter 6

Feeding problems and their treatment

Gillian Harris, *University of Birmingham*

There are two areas in infancy that are usually perceived as 'feeding' problems; these are the refusal or inability to take in food orally, or growth faltering where there is no associated underlying organic disease. Obesity as a result of taking in too much food is not usually perceived in itself to be a problem in infancy, although it might be thought to be a risk factor for later life.

The refusal to take food can also be described or further subdivided in various ways. The infant might take too little food, that is, too few calories to maintain optimal growth or, once solid foods have been introduced, might take such a restricted range of foods that dietary balance is compromised. Alternatively, the infant's feeding behaviour might be seen as problematic. One such behavioural problem is likely to be that of slow feeding, taking in very small amounts of food over a prolonged period. The infant might also show avoidance or negative behaviours, such as crying and headturning, at mealtimes. More severe behaviours might also occur which preclude the swallowing or digestion of food. These might include holding food in the mouth, regurgitating and ruminating, spitting, gagging or vomiting. Finally, children might be perceived as having feeding problems because they lack appropriate oral–motor feeding skills, such as swallowing, sucking or moving food appropriately around the mouth.

Growth faltering is likely to be perceived as a feeding problem where negative feeding behaviours, lack of feeding skills, or a loss of appetite are perceived as the reason for an insufficient calorie intake. Where growth faltering in infancy has no organic base, then the relationship between the infant and the mother, the person usually responsible for feeding the child, is often called into question. But such growth faltering, usually termed non-organic failure to thrive, can still be best described as a failure to take in sufficient calories for optimal growth (Whitten *et al.*, 1969). Whether this reduced intake is due to factors within the child, factors within the mother, or the mismanagement of the child's feeding regime, is still a matter of debate.

Although weight faltering is more likely to be perceived specifically as a feeding problem where there is no known organic cause, feeding difficulties can still occur as secondary to known medical conditions. However, these difficulties can still best be described as either problems of intake, problems associated with feeding behaviours or problems associated with a lack of feeding skills.

We can also divide feeding problems according to the age of the infant. Problems of early infancy are likely to be those of refusal to suck at the breast or bottle, slow or prolonged feeding and inadequate intake. Further difficulties might be caused by vomiting or regurgitating feeds. During the transitional period, at approximately three months of age, when the infant is being introduced to solid foods then the problem of restricted intake might become apparent. Infants might either refuse to take any solid foods or will only take a very limited range of tastes or textures, with most of their calories coming from milk. As the child's autonomy and mobility increase during the first and into the second year, then so does the likelihood of extreme faddiness or of negative feeding behaviours occurring. Growth faltering also becomes more apparent as the infant gets older and comparisons are made with standardised centile charts. Therefore, concern about the long-term consequences of poor intake is also likely to increase during the first year.

Non-organic failure to thrive

A working definition of non-organic failure to thrive is of weight faltering down across centile lines to a point below the third centile on standardised weight charts. Weight faltering would have to last for a period longer than six months with onset typically at three or nine months of age. Such weight faltering would also have to occur in the absence of any organic disease which might explain such loss. The explanation for such weight faltering, and therefore the main focus for intervention, has typically been the relationship between mother and infant. The historical precedent for such assumption of causality can be traced back to early observation of infants placed in institutions who failed to thrive, and often died (Gardner, 1972). The cause was not seen to be lack of stimulation, but lack of maternal 'warmth'. Gardner (1972) wrote 'It has long been known that infants will not thrive if their mothers are hostile to them or even merely indifferent.' This assumption has meant that for many years intervention programmes aimed at children with weight faltering have been directed at the general relationship between mother and infant. Only recently has research looked specifically at feeding interactions, and been directed at an understanding of the regulators of appetite and food choice in infancy.

Non-organic failure to thrive has been termed 'emotional abuse' (Iwaniec *et al.*, 1988) and the mechanisms within the child that result in failure to thrive have been seen as akin to those of anaclictic depression (Spitz, 1946). As a result of insufficient stimulation by the mother or of lack of response by the mother to the infant's overtures, the infant of a depressed, withdrawn or unresponsive mother withdraws, becoming in turn socially unresponsive. This withdrawal was thought to lead either to loss of appetite within the infant or to cause growth retardation through the mediation of hormonal inactivity (Gardner, 1972). Some attempts have been made to separate out these two conditions, loss of appetite and hormonally mediated growth retardation, and term them non-organic failure to thrive and deprivation dwarfism, respectively. In the latter syndrome, deprivation dwarfism, infants show later onset of growth faltering and of feeding difficulties, and there is evidence of growth hormone deficiency (Oates, 1984). Whilst attempting to differentiate between the two syndromes, however, Oates found evidence that similar home environments, that of chaotic deprivation, were common to both groups of children. This might seem to suggest that failure to thrive could be seen merely in terms of infant neglect. What is not clear however is, if non-organic failure to thrive is to be seen as a function of maternal state, or of home environment, why only some children of depressed or disorganised mothers fail to thrive. Indeed, within large families, in which all the children are similarly neglected, only one child may fail to thrive. It would seem that there is not a linear causal relationship between maternal, or environmental, factors and failure to thrive, but that these add to cumulative risk factors for any one specific child. It might be that some children are inherently more difficult to feed than others (Pollitt, 1973; Derivan, 1982), due either to the child's past experience with food, or due to a dysfunction in the regulation of appetite. If this were true it might also be that mothers of children who refuse to feed become depressed, or anxious, because of the difficulties entailed in attempting to feed a child without appetite.

Further differentiation within the non-organic failure to thrive population was suggested by Linscheid and Rasnake (1986) who described two distinct stages of failure to thrive. The first, Type I, has its onset in the first few months of life. Interaction between the mother–infant dyad is generally poor and the syndrome is described as an attachment disorder; a failure in the formation of a relationship between mother and infant (Benoit *et al.*, 1989). The second classification, Type II, is described as a separation disorder; the mother does not allow the infant to take control over his or her own behaviour. In the Type II classification, the onset of feeding problems is not usually observed until the second year of life, and problems in the relationship between mother and infant do not extend beyond mealtimes. The behaviours described in the Type II classification, rooted hypothetically in the onset of toddler autonomy (Chatoor *et al.*, 1985), are however very frequently observed in clinical populations of children where there is a known organic disorder (Harris and Booth, 1992), and could be better described as chronic food refusal.

In a study by Skuse *et al.* (1992), comparing interactions between mothers of infants with failure to thrive and matched controls and where socio-economic status of the mother was held constant, no difference was found between the two groups in incidence of depression or other psychopathology. Mothers of infants with failure to thrive did, however, get fewer calories into the infant than did mothers of control group infants (although sufficient may have been offered) and did use maladaptive feeding management techniques; the infants frequently showed food-refusing behaviour. Similar patterns of parental behaviour are found where failure to thrive is associated with a known organic disorder. In a study by Harris and Macdonald (1992), feeding problems in the child were related to high anxiety levels in the parent. Pre-school children with cystic fibrosis, a condition in which children need to have a high calorie intake in order to maintain optimal lung function, were assessed for the nature and extent of their feeding problems and compared with a matched control group. In the cystic fibrosis group, where parental anxiety about intake was high, children were more likely to show negative behaviours at mealtimes, and parents were more likely to use coercive or forceful management techniques to get the children to eat.

It would seem therefore that the distinction between non-organic failure to thrive and failure to thrive with associated organic disorder is a difficult one to make. Infants initially diagnosed as non-organic failure to thrive are often found to have an associated organic disorder (Benoit *et al.*, 1989). This organic disorder is not usually thought by itself to be serious enough to warrant growth faltering, but in interaction with other factors must contribute to the feeding problem. We cannot therefore assume that the categories of failure to thrive, non-organic failure to thrive, and food refusal describe discrete populations of infants. The aetiologies of failure to thrive are many and multi-factorial. The mode of treatment must therefore be individually tailored to the infant and family, with observations and assessment of parental style of interaction, mode of mealtime management and history of the infant's feeding behaviour all being taken into consideration.

Treatment

In addressing these feeding problems, i.e. growth faltering and the inability or refusal to take food, five intervention models are usually employed: the physiological, the behavioural, the interactional, the cognitive and the mechanical. The physiological model looks at the development of the acquisition of self-regulation of appetite and is directed at understanding the nature of possible dysfunction within the infant. The behavioural model is based upon the assumption that food refusal is due to learned responses, usually conditioned aversions to negative feeding experiences. Behavioural interventions are primarily directed at the management of feeding behaviours and aim to increase intake by concentrating upon external constraints to feeding. The interactional model is based upon the assumption that feeding behaviour and intake, and hence growth, will improve if the relationship between mother, as primary caregiver, and infant is enhanced. The cognitive model stresses the child's understanding of processes involved in the formation of food preferences or in appetite regulation, and is therefore usually applicable only to older children. However, imitative behaviour, which might be subsumed in this model, is observed even in infancy. The mechanical model addresses such issues as feeding position on breast or teat in early infancy, and the acquisition of oral–motor skills in later infancy.

These intervention models differ therefore in their emphasis; they are concerned either with the management of skills or behaviours, and concentrate either on the infant or the mother as the causal agent in the feeding problem.

Physiological models

One important finding which could be incorporated into future intervention studies with specific populations where non-organic failure to thrive is prevalent is that such failure to thrive is related to the age of the introduction of solid foods to the infant. This concept of a sensitive period for the introduction of solid foods was first suggested by Illingworth and Lister (1964) and now seems to be supported by a study carried out on an urban population where non-organic failure to thrive was rife (Fell et al., 1992). Within this population, weight faltering and poor feeding skills were found to be associated with the delay of the introduction of solid foods until late in the first year.

The mean age of introduction of solid foods by middle-class breast- and bottle-feeding urban mothers is approximately fourteen weeks (Harris, 1988). Mothers within these populations usually introduced solids because they observed a change in infant behaviour which they interpreted as increased hunger. The changes which they observed were usually of renewed night waking or more frequent feeding. At around this same age, from three to four months, there seems to be a period of optimal acceptance of different tastes which might be offered to the infant (Harris et al., 1990). After this seemingly sensitive period taste preferences are determined merely by exposure (Beauchamp and Moran, 1984). That is, in children as in adults, taste preferences are learned by experiencing the specific taste or the specific food. However, as infants get older, they become more conservative about the foods that they will either eat or try for the first time (Birch and Marlin, 1982; Harris and Booth, 1987). It is probably safe to assume therefore that the later the introduction of solid foods, the more difficult the introduction is likely to become.

Another component of appetite regulation that is learned is the timing of meals (Weingarten, 1983). Adults learn to be hungry at the time at which they normally eat. If adults wish to lose weight then the most reliable strategy is to cut out snacks in between main meals (Booth, 1988). However, a strategy still prevalent in the management of failure to thrive in infants and young children is to feed the child large but infrequent meals, so that the child might become hungry. Infrequent low-calorie meals are in fact implicated in failure to thrive (Pugliese *et al.*, 1987), and some treatment models therefore suggest offering small and frequent meals (Harris and Booth, 1992).

Difficulties also arise when attempting to supplement a child's intake with calorie-dense additives or by naso-gastric feeding. The regulation of calorie intake has been shown to operate in children of two to five years (Birch *et al.*, 1991) and the onset of this process has been discussed in an earlier chapter (chapter 4). Infants will regulate their milk intake, although this regulation is not absolute, in that calorie intake will be modified towards an approximation of normal intake (Fomon *et al.*, 1975). The addition of calorie-dense supplements, or the implementation of naso-gastric feeding to improve weight gain in infants with failure to thrive, although useful in the short term (Ramsey and Zelazo, 1988) may be maladaptive in the longer term. The continued use of feeding supplementation, given that the child will move towards calorie regulation, means that oral feeding may be further reduced, and naso-gastric feeding becomes the main source of intake (Geertsma *et al.*, 1985). This is likely to happen more frequently where the child has behavioural feeding difficulties, or a dysfunction in oral–motor skills. Parents who have to feed the child avoid the more difficult option, that of feeding the child orally, and also come to rely upon the naso-gastric feed.

Although no work has yet been carried out on the relationship between a developmental delay in the ability to regulate appetite, and growth and feeding disorders, it seems feasible that there might be a causal link. Certainly, many children with failure to thrive also have speech disorders (Skuse, 1992), which might seem to indicate the presence of some specific learning difficulties as well as possible oral–motor dysfunction. Those infants who cannot regulate intake to accord with growth velocity, who do not feel hunger or perhaps just do not signal hunger, might well be at risk of later feeding disorders. Skuse *et al.* (1992) have noted that infants with failure to thrive are often perceived as 'easy' to feed in that they make few demands upon the parent. They do not cry frequently for food and can be left for long periods without feeding (Evans and Davies, 1977).

Behavioural models

Both faddiness and food refusal can be thought of as learned responses to avoid negative consequences. The pairing of nausea or vomiting with the ingestion of food can cause subsequent avoidance of that food whether or not the food has caused the vomiting (Rozin, 1986). Thus many infants, either on aversive drug regimes, or with oesophagial reflux, are likely to avoid foods that have been paired with nausea in the past. Similarly, if mealtimes are tense and angry affairs accompanied by threats and force-feeding, then the infant will learn to avoid or show avoidance behaviours at the sight of food or feeding equipment. In addition, parents frequently manage to reinforce unwanted behaviours by attending more to incidences of food refusal than to incidences of food acceptance. Behavioural programmes are therefore best implemented where the infant has found mealtimes or food aversive, and where it is necessary to pair feeding behaviour with pleasant stimuli and to give positive reinforcement of appropriate feeding behaviour.

Behavioural intervention programmes are usually reported as studies on specific patient populations (Linscheid *et al.*, 1987; Blackman and Nelson, 1985; Palmer *et al.*, 1975; Geertsma *et al.*, 1985; Handen *et al.*, 1986; Bernal, 1972; Larson *et al.*, 1987; Singer *et al.*, 1991). Such programmes are usually carried out as single or multiple case studies and as such usually entail no control condition. They are based on reinforcement of appropriate feeding behaviour, whilst hoping for extinction of negative or incompatible behaviours. Such intervention programmes were perhaps used most widely in the 1970s with adolescents diagnosed as having anorexia nervosa. In these programmes the consumption of a set calorie intake would be reinforced with specific privileges. Similar intervention programmes are now used with in-patient populations of children showing food refusal and failure to thrive, usually associated with an underlying disease process which affects appetite or weight gain. Frequently the intervention programmes are designed to change the children's feeding regimes from naso-gastric to oral feeds (Geertsma *et al.*, 1985; Blackman and Nelson, 1985); most effect some degree of change. Programmes have been reported as being successful with children aged 10 to 40 months with failure to thrive secondary to cystic fibrosis (Singer *et al.*, 1991), and with infants aged 4 to 21 months showing failure to thrive associated with diagnosed physiological disorders (Larson *et al.*, 1987). Children were included in these intervention programmes because of weight faltering associated with poor calorie intake, and because of negative behaviour at mealtimes. Negative behaviours included strong avoidance responses at mealtimes, as well as spitting, gagging and vomiting. Reinforcement on these programmes was either paired with appropriate eating behaviour (attention, praise or music); or contingent upon appropriate eating behaviour (stickers, toy-play or television). Time out was used to achieve extinction of inappropriate behaviours and was defined as averting eye contact or removing the infant from the stimulus environment for short periods. Three of the four children with cystic fibrosis showed improved intake and growth, although it is not clear which part of the programme was most effective. Similarly, all three of the infants in the Larson study showed increased food acceptance and decreases in negative behaviours. However, as none of these intervention programmes used control comparisons, it could of course be that inclusion in an intervention programme in itself brings about an improvement in feeding behaviour.

Improvements in feeding behaviour have also been reported for studies using coercive methods of reintroducing oral feeding. Palmer *et al.* (1975), using a behavioural intervention model, reported that a distressed child was ignored for three hours until some food had been taken. Blackman and Nelson (1985) also advocate firm management in which 'feedings continue despite initial resistance'. This programme of forcible feeding is reported as reintroducing ten out of eleven failure-to-thrive tube-fed children to oral feeding during a three-week period. However, no follow-up data are provided for this study. Similarly, aversive techniques have been used to treat rumination in infants (Cunningham and Linscheid, 1976). Such aversive programmes are not, however, likely to establish normal positive feeding behaviours in the home environment. In fact, force-feeding by the parent is usually a precursor to food refusal by the child (Harris and Booth, 1992).

Interactional models

Models of intervention based on changing the nature of the interaction between the caregiver (usually the mother) and infant are based on one of two assumptions. The first is that maternal state of mind (depression, anxiety) will affect her relationship with her infant and that this in turn will affect the feeding interaction; the second is that the mother's lack of skill in managing the infant, or insensitivity to the infant's needs, will determine the infant's ultimate calorie intake. Where mothers themselves have feeding disorders, it has also been suggested that the nature of the disorder distorts the mother's perception of her infant's feeding behaviour, or increases the amount of control that the mother attempts to place on the feeding interaction (Stein, personal communication).

A recent study by Hellin and Waller (1992) showed that mothers who scored highly on the Beck Depression Inventory during pregnancy were more likely to report physical difficulties when breast-feeding their infants, and to give up breast-feeding sooner, than women who were not depressed. Mothers who were rated as more anxious a week after delivery tended to perceive their infants as more fussy. High anxiety ratings after birth were also related to the early introduction of solids and concern over the infant's calorie intake. Where mothers are more anxious about intake they are more likely to override infant signals of satiety in order to get the infant to take more food (Harris and Macdonald, 1992). If an infant's behavioural signals of satiety have been ignored by an anxious or insensitive parent attempting to impose control over infant intake, then the strength of such signals will be increased by the infant (Harris and Booth, 1992). The infant then has to indicate satiety by screaming, head turning or vomiting. Parents who are unable to respond sensitively to infant signals may also ignore signals of hunger, such as movements towards the spoon or bowl, or mouth–opening responses. By educating parents to recognise and respond appropriately to infant signals of hunger and satiety, negative behaviours need no longer be expressed by the infant. However, in such an intervention study aimed at increasing oral intake for five infants aged five to nine months (Ramsey and Zelazo, 1988), it was observed that a programme designed to improve interaction at mealtimes between mother and infant resulted in greater shifts in infant social behaviour than in maternal social behaviour. This increase co-varied with increased acceptance of bottle-feeding.

It seems that much of the success of interactionally based programmes might be in the cessation of force-feeding and the desensitisation of the infant to aversive stimuli. However, it is also important to educate parents to respond sensitively to infant behavioural signals of hunger and satiety, especially as infants with failure to thrive seem to perform poorly on measures of non-verbal communicative skill (Skuse *et al.*, 1992).

Some intervention programmes for children who refuse to feed, or who show growth faltering, are aimed not at improving specific aspects of the interaction between mother and infant, but at improving the general relationship between the two, or of family functioning as a whole. Iwaniec and Herbert (1982) dealt with the mother's feelings of anger towards the child, or the level of 'emotional arousal between mother and child', with a multi-stage but non-specific 'supportive' intervention programme. An 82 per cent success rate was given for this programme but no baseline or follow-up data were given. The criterion of success was discharge from social work care.

Cognitive models

The studies in this area are usually based upon research into regulators of intake and food preference in children within a normal population. Such studies that have been carried out have also usually looked at the modification of food preference in pre-school children rather than in infants. However, the findings can be applied to children in their second year, when most problems of food refusal become more acute.

Two studies show the importance of imitation on children's willingness to try new foods. The first study carried out by Harper and Sanders (1975) looked at the effect of modelling on the behaviour of children from the age of fourteen months. Children of this age are more likely to try a novel food if they first see an adult, but not necessarily the parent, taste the food. It is interesting to note here that an intervention study that appears to support the efficacy of a behavioural approach to the increase of food consumption in a child does in fact on closer reading demonstrate the use of parental modelling. Bernal (1972) reported a behavioural programme carried out with a four-year-old girl, in which an attempt to increase the child's consumption of adult food, by allowing her to watch television, was unsuccessful. The child did, however, start to eat adult food when she asked for and ate a portion of her father's breakfast cereal; this behaviour was retained although it was not directly reinforced.

With older children it might seem that peer group modelling is more important. Birch (1980), working with pre-school children, showed that preference for foods previously rated by a child as neutral could be increased if the child was seated during a mealtime with other children whose rating of that food was higher. Both consumption and rating of the target food were observed to increase, and this increase was maintained at a re-test.

In similar studies (Birch *et al.*, 1982; Newman and Taylor, 1992; Lepper *et al.*, 1982) it was found that children's preferences were affected by their perception of the 'value' of a food. For example, where consumption of one food is made contingent upon consumption of another food (eat up A and then you can have B), the instrumental food (A) was consequently devalued and consumption decreased. Consumption and preference rating of the reward food (B), however, increased. These findings are of relevance to those who would adopt a behavioural intervention model. By rewarding a child for eating specific foods, or specific calorie loads, it would seem that either eating *per se*, or eating specific foods, would be devalued. It would also seem to mitigate against using the consumption of 'undesirable' foods (sweets, puddings) as a reward for the consumption of 'desirable' foods (vegetables).

Careful reading of the literature suggests that it is better to use an intervention model involving classical conditioning, that is, pairing eating with some form of reinforcing agent (Birch *et al.*, 1980) rather than to adopt an operant conditioning paradigm; making reward contingent upon food consumption. Although the latter might work in the short term, it would seem to have negative effects in the long term on children's cognitions about food and eating.

Mechanical models

Given that most infants with failure to thrive will gain weight if they are hospitalised and fed naso-gastrically (Goldbloom, 1982), weight faltering is increasingly defined as a problem of poor calorie intake (Bell and Woolston, 1985), rather than as a problem of growth retardation given sufficient calorie intake. Poor calorie intake may be a function of oral–motor dysfunction or swallowing difficulties, which may lead to aspiration of the food (Evans-Morris, 1977). If the child is unable to process the food adequately through the mouth then feeding will be slow and difficult for both child and parent. In these situations parents are apt to give up rather too quickly on the feeding process. Children with some specific disorders may find eating difficult because of poor positioning, or seating arrangements at mealtimes (Crane,

1987). Reilly and Skuse (1992) studied a group of 12 children aged 15–39 months with cerebral palsy and compared their feeding behaviour with that of a matched control group. They found that failure to thrive was more common in the children with cerebral palsy, and was associated with short mealtimes, poor positioning at mealtimes and greater oral–motor dysfunction. Such problems cause difficulty not only because they prolong mealtimes and reduce intake, but also because in cases where food is aspirated or where choking follows swallowing difficulties, feeding becomes aversive to the child.

Many treatment schedules directed at problems with breast-feeding in early infancy deal mainly with 'mechanical' issues, such as the positioning of the mouth on the nipple or positioning of the infant's head to allow respiration However, there is the suggestion (Bu'lock et al., 1990) that infants' refusal to feed even at the breast might be related to an acquired conditioned aversion. In an attempt to resolve positioning problems whilst breast-feeding the infant might be forcibly pushed onto the breast, thus making breast-feeding aversive to the infant. Wooldridge has suggested (personal communication) that the way in which such a problem of breast refusal is best resolved is by allowing the infant to take control and regulate the pattern of breast feeds, even if this means frequent breaks to the feed.

Conclusion

There have been many, usually small-scale, studies directed at the improvement of children's feeding behaviour. Most of these studies have a behavioural component and most of them report some degree of success in terms of weight gain or increase in calorie intake. However, few studies use any form of control condition, so it is never quite clear which component of the treatment package is effective. Often treatment components are confounded with other variables, as in the study by Bernal (1972), thus making the effective component even more difficult to isolate.

Those intervention studies that have been directed at improving nutritional status and increasing growth by improving the style of interaction between parent and child do not usually look closely at the infant's feeding behaviour to see if food refusal is implicated. Therefore we often do not know whether programmes directed at changing the relationship between mother and infant (Herbert, 1987) are in fact having greater effect on the behaviour of the infant (Ramsey and Zelazo, 1988). It is also difficult to make comparisons in the efficacy of intervention programmes because of differences between studies in inclusion criteria, the ages of the infants studied, and the severity of weight faltering. One study (Drotar et al., 1985) does make a comparison between types of treatment. However, although all intervention programmes studied were successful in outcome, no one type of treatment was found to be more successful than the others. It would seem that any type of intervention works equally well.

Further problems are caused by the attempts made to subdivide growth failure and problems of intake into discrete categories of non-organic and organic failure to thrive, and to assume that all cases of non-organic failure to thrive are due only to problems in the relationship between infant and mother. It would be more useful in terms of treatment modalities to assume that all cases of failure to thrive are due to reduced or restricted calorie intake by the child, and that such a poor calorie intake may be based on many factors. Such factors include the infant's ability to regulate appetite and intake, the infant's ability to communicate hunger and satiety, the parent's ability to respond appropriately to those signals of hunger and satiety when feeding the infant, the infant's past experiences with feeding, and the infant's actual skill and ability in sucking, chewing or swallowing food. In feeding disorders both with or without observable organic cause there may be problems in any or all of these areas. This does not mean that the parent's mood does not affect infant feeding behaviour and appetite regulation. For example, a parent who is depressed may not respond to an infant's signals of hunger, especially if those signals are weak, and the infant might fail to be given sufficient calories. A parent who is anxious about the infant's nutritional status because of a known organic problem may well override the infant's signals of satiety and force-feed. In both these cases the parent is not able to help the infant towards the successful regulation and integration of appetite, intake and growth; a successful regulation which is based on the social reinforcement ensuing from a stress-free feeding interaction.

We could perhaps think of feeding, and consequently growth problems, in simplistic terms, as ranged along a continuum of self-regulatory ability. Those infants who show a delay in regulatory ability are at risk of failure to thrive if paired with parents who are unable or unwilling to respond to weak behavioural signals, or who do not provide a structured regime of feeds for the infant. At the other end of the continuum lie infants with strong behavioural signals of hunger and satiety with parents who are trying to control intake for the infant, and therefore override their self-regulatory system. Intervention packages must therefore take account of both infant behaviour and the way in which this interacts with parental style of management.

References

Beauchamp, G.K. and Moran, M. (1984), 'Acceptance of sweet and salty tastes in 2-year-old children', *Appetite*, 5, pp. 291–305.

Bell, L.S. and Woolston, J.L. (1985), 'The relationship of weight gain and calorie intake in infants with organic and non-organic failure to thrive syndrome', *Journal of the American Academy of Child Psychiatry*, 24, pp. 447–52.

Benoit, D., Zeanah, C. and Barton, M. (1989), 'Maternal attachment disturbances in failure to thrive', *Infant Mental Health Journal*, 10, pp. 185–202.

Bernal, M. (1972), 'Behavioural treatment of a child's eating problem', *Journal of Behavioural Therapy and Experimental Psychiatry*, 3, pp. 43–50.

Birch, L.L. (1980), 'Effects of peer models' food choice and eating behaviors on preschoolers food preferences', *Child Development*, 51, pp. 489–96.

Birch, L.L., Johnson, S.L., Andersen, G., Peters, J.C. and Schulte, M.C. (1991), 'The variability of young children's energy intake', *New England Journal of Medicine*, 324, pp. 232–5.

Birch, L.L. and Marlin, D.W. (1982), 'Eating as a "means" activity in a contingency: effects on young children's food preference', *Child Development*, 55, pp. 431–9.

Birch, L.L., Marlin, D.W. and Rotter, J. (1984), 'I don't like it, I never tried it: effects of exposure to food on two-year-old children's food preferences', *Appetite*, 3, pp. 353–60.

Birch, L.L., Zimmerman, S.I. and Hind, H. (1980), 'The influence of social-effective context on the formation of children's food preferences', *Child Development*, 51, pp. 856–61.

Blackman, J.A. and Nelson, C.L. (1985), 'Reinstituting oral feedings in children fed by gastromony tube', *Clinical Pediatrics*, 24, pp. 434–8.

Booth, D.A. (1988), 'Mechanisms from models – actual effects from real life: the zero-calorie drink break option', *Appetite*, 11, *Supplement*, pp. 94–102.

Bu'lock, F., Wooldridge, M.W. and Baum, J.D. (1990), 'Development of coordination of sucking, swallowing and breathing. Ultrasound study of term and pre-term infants', *Developmental Medicine and Child Neurology*, 32, pp. 669–78.

Chatoor, I., Dickson, L., Schaefer, S. and Egan, J. (1985), 'A developmental classification of feeding disorders associated with failure to thrive: diagnosis and treatment', in D. Drotar (ed.), *New Directions in Failure to Thrive: Implications for research and practice*, (New York: Plenum).

Crane, S. (1987), 'Feeding the handicapped child – a review of intervention strategies', *Nutrition and Health*, 5, pp. 109–18.

Cunningham, C.E. and Linscheid, T.R. (1976), 'Elimination of chronic infant ruminating by electric shock', *Behaviour Therapy*, 7, pp. 231–4.

Derivan, A.T. (1982), 'Disorders of bonding', in P.J. Accardo (ed.), *Failure to Thrive in Infancy and Early Childhood: A multi-disciplinary approach* (Baltimore, MD; University Park Press).

Drotar, D., Nowak, M., Malone, C.A., Eckerle, D. and Negray, J. (1985), 'Early psychological outcomes in failure to thrive: predictions from an interactional model', *Journal of Clinical Child Psychology*, 14, pp. 105–11.

Evans, T.J. and Davies, D.P. (1977), 'Failure to thrive at the breast: an old problem revisited', *Archives of Disease in Childhood*, 52, p. 947.

Evans-Morris, S. (1977), 'Oral–motor development: normal and abnormal', in J.M. Wilson (ed.), *Oral Motor Function and Dysfunction in Children* (Chapel Hill, NC: University of North Carolina).

Fell, J., Debelle, G., Macdonald, A., Harris, G. and Booth, I.W. (1992), 'Early childhood feeding practices and nutritional status of Asian children in Central Birmingham', in preparation.

Fomon, S.J., Filer, L.J., Thomas, L.N., Anderson, T.A. and Nelson, S.E. (1975), 'Influence of formula concentration on caloric intake and growth of normal infants', *Acta Paediatrica Scandinavica*, 64, pp. 172–81.

Gardner, L.I. (1972), 'Deprivation dwarfism', in *Readings from Scientific American: The nature and nurture of behavior* (San Francisco: Freeman).

Geertsma, M.A., Hyams, J.S., Pelletier, J.M. and Reiters, S. (1985), 'Feeding resistance after parenteral hyperalimentation', *American Journal of Diseases in Childhood*, **139**, pp. 255–6.

Goldbloom, R.B. (1982), 'Failure to thrive', *Pediatric Clinics of North America*, **29**, pp. 151–66.

Handen, B., Mandell, F. and Russo, D. (1986), 'Feeding induction in children who refuse to eat', *American Journal of Diseases in Childhood*, **140**, pp. 52–4.

Harper, L. and Sanders, K. (1975), 'The effect of adult's eating on young children's acceptance of unfamiliar foods', *Journal of Experimental Child Psychology*, **20**, pp. 206–14.

Harris, G. (1988), 'Determinants of the introduction of solid food', *Journal of Reproductive and Infant Psychology*, **6**, pp. 241–9.

Harris, G. and Booth, D.A. (1987), 'Infant's preference for salt in food: its dependence upon recent dietary experience', *Journal of Reproductive and Infant Psychology*, **5**, pp. 97–104.

Harris, G. and Booth, I.W. (1992), 'The nature and management of eating problems in pre-school children', in P. Cooper and A. Stein (eds), *Monographs in Clinical Pediatrics, Vol. 5, Feeding problems and eating disorders in children and adolescents* (Chur, Switzerland: Harwood).

Harris, G. and Macdonald, A. (1992), 'Behavioural feeding problems in cystic fibrosis', Paper given at the Sixth Annual Cystic Fibrosis Conference, Washington, DC.

Harris, G., Thomas, A.M. and Booth, D.A. (1990), 'Development of salt taste in infancy', *Developmental Psychology*, **268**, pp. 535–8.

Hellin, K. and Waller, G. (1992), 'Mothers' mood and infant feeding: predictions of problems and practices', *Journal of Reproductive and Infant Psychology*, **10**, pp. 39–51.

Herbert, M. (1987), *Behavioural Treatment of Children with Problems: A practice manual* (London: Academic).

Illingworth, R.S. and Lister, J. (1964), 'The critical or sensitive period with specific reference to certain feeding problems in infants and children', *Journal of Pediatrics*, **65**, pp. 839–84.

Iwaniec, D. and Herbert, M. (1982), 'The assessment and treatment of children who fail to thrive', *Social Work Today*, **13**, pp. 8–12.

Iwaniec, D., Herbert, M. and Sluckin, A. (1988), 'Helping emotionally abused children who fail to thrive', in K. Browne, C. Davies and P. Stratton (eds), *Early Prediction and Prevention of Child Abuse* (Chichester: John Wiley).

Larson, K., Allyon, T. and Barrett, D. (1987), 'A behavioural feeding program for failure to thrive infants', *Behavioural Research and Therapy*, **25**, pp. 39–47.

Lepper, M., Sagotsky, G., Dafoe, J. and Greene, D. (1982), 'Consequences of superfluous social constraints on young children's social inferences and subsequent intrinsic interest', *Journal of Personality and Social Psychology*, **2**, pp. 51–65.

Linscheid, T.R. and Rasnake, L.K. (1986), 'Behavioral approaches to the treatment of failure to thrive', in D. Drotar (ed.), *New Directions in Failure to Thrive: Implications for research and practice* (New York: Plenum).

Linscheid, T.R., Tarnowski, K.J., Rasnake, L.K. and Brams, J.S. (1987), 'Behavioral treatment of food refusal in a child with short-gut syndrome', *Journal of Pediatric Psychology*, **12**, pp. 451–9.

Newman, J. and Taylor, A. (1992), 'Effects of a means–end contingency on young children's food preferences', *Journal of Experimental Child Psychology*, **64**, pp. 200–16.

Oates, R.K. (1984), 'Similarities and differences between nonorganic failure to thrive and deprivation dwarfism', *Child Abuse and Neglect*, 8, pp. 439–45.

Palmer, S., Thompson, R.J. and Linscheid, T.R. (1975), 'Applied behaviour analysis in the treatment of childhood feeding problems', *Developmental Medicine and Child Neurology*, 17, pp. 333–9.

Pollitt, E. (1973), 'Behavior of infants in causation of nutritional marasmus', *American Journal of Clinical Nutrition*, 26, pp. 264–70.

Pugliese, M.T., Weyman-Daum, M., Moses, N. and Lifshitz, F. (1987), 'Parental health beliefs as a cause of nonorganic failure to thrive', *Pediatrics*, 80, pp. 175–82.

Ramsey, M. and Zelazo, P. (1988), 'Food refusal in failure to thrive infants; nasogastric feeding combined with interactive-behavioural treatment', *Journal of Pediatric Psychology*, 13, pp. 329–47.

Reilly, S. and Skuse, D. (1992), 'Characteristics and management of feeding problems of young children with cerebral palsy', *Developmental Medicine and Child Neorology*, 34, pp. 379–88.

Rozin, P. (1986), 'One trial acquired likes and dislikes in humans; disgust as a US, food predominance and negative learning predominance', *Learning and Motivation*, 17, pp. 180–9.

Singer, L.T., Nofer, J.A., Benson-Szekely, L.J. and Brooks, L.J. (1991), 'Behavioral assessment and management of food refusal in children with cystic fibrosis', *Developmental and Behavioral Pediatrics*, 12, pp. 115–19.

Skuse, D. (1992), 'The relationship between deprivation, physical growth and the impaired development of language', in P. Fletcher (ed.), *Proceedings of the 2nd International Symposium Specific Speech and Language Disorders in Children* (London: Whurr).

Skuse, D., Wolke, D. and Reilly, S. (1992), 'Failure to thrive: clinical and developmental aspects', in H. Remschmidt and M. Schmidt (eds), *Child and Youth Psychiatry: European Perspectives. Vol. II: Developmental psychopathology* (Lewiston: Hogrefe and Huber).

Spitz, R.A. (1946), 'Anaclitic depression', *Psychoanalytic Study of the Child*, 2, pp. 313–42.

Weingarten, H.P. (1983), 'Conditioned cues elicit feeding in sated rats: a role for learning in meal initiation', *Science*, 220, pp. 431–3.

Whitten, C.F., Pettit, M.G. and Fischoff, J. (1969), 'Evidence that growth failure from maternal deprivation is secondary to under-eating', *Journal of the American Medical Association*, 209, pp. 1675–82.

Part 3

Sleeping

Chapter 7

The physiology of sleep in infants and young children

Zenobia Zaiwalla, *Park Hospital for Children, Oxford,*
and Alan Stein, *University of Oxford*

Introduction

Sleep is a reversible behavioural state of perceptual disengagement from and
reduced responsiveness to the environment. It is a complex amalgam of
physiological and behavioural processes accompanied by characteristic EEG
changes (Carskadon and Dement, 1989).

At the beginning of this century wakefulness was thought to be maintained
by continuous sensory input to the brain (Kleitman and Camille, 1932) and
thought to depend on the intactness of sensory pathways to the brain. In 1949,
Moruzzi and Magoun demonstrated that the electrical stimulation of the
brainstem reticular formation produced cortical activation in an otherwise
sleeping animal preparation. Once this concept of an activating system
maintaining wakefulness was accepted, sleep was thought to be due to fatigue
of this system, suggesting a passive process (Moruzzi, 1972). However,
transectional studies in animals soon demonstrated the existence of sleep-
generating structures in the lower brainstem. In the last fifty years the basic
mechanisms of the sleep/wake cycle have been studied by a multidisciplinary
approach including neurophysiology, neuroanatomy and neurochemistry.
What has emerged from these studies is that a neuronal system which governs
cyclic alteration between waking and sleep is situated in the core of the brain
extending from the medulla through the brainstem and hypothalamus into the
forebrain (Jones, 1989). No single group of neurons is uniquely involved in
maintaining one state, although there is possibly a differential concentration
of cells mainly responsible for wakefulness and those mainly involved in
inducing and maintaining sleep, with close links between the neuronal groups.

In order to understand the physiology of sleep in infants, it is important first to describe sleep in normal adults. This is because most of the original research into the physiology of sleep was done using adult subjects and the physiological and behavioural features of sleep in adulthood are more stable and easily defined. Thus this chapter will begin with a description of sleep architecture, the progression of sleep across the night and changes in other physiological parameters which accompany sleep in adults. This is then followed by a description of the physiological development and distribution of sleep patterns in neonates and infants, including the development of REM/non-REM sleep, the sleep/wake cycle, as well as changes in other physiological parameters accompanying sleep as they differ from adults and older children. EEG and sleep patterns in infancy as possible predictors of later intellectual development are then discussed. Finally, some of the theories of the function of sleep are considered.

Normal sleep physiology

Sleep architecture

Within sleep, two different states have been recognised. They are the non-rapid-eye-movement (NREM) state and the rapid-eye-movement (REM) state (Rechtschaffen and Kales, 1968). The recognition of these two states is based on defined criteria of changes in physiological parameters including EEG (electroencephalogram), muscle tone (EMG (electromyogram)) and eye movements.

NREM sleep is conventionally divided into four stages (Carskadon and Dement, 1989). Stages one and two are light sleep stages, while stages three and four represent deep sleep with a high arousal threshold. The EEG characteristics of NREM sleep include phasic events like spindles and K complexes superimposed on a background of high-voltage synchronous slow waves.[1] The K complexes represent an internal arousal system and are more prominent in stage two sleep than in deep sleep. They may be followed by a brief arousal, sometimes accompanied by a limb jerk. NREM sleep is ontogenically younger and is characteristic of mammalian and avian sleep and is thought to have evolved with the homeothermic (warm-blooded) state.

REM sleep, also called active sleep or paradoxical sleep, is ontogenically primitive sleep and is characterised by EEG activation not unlike the wake state, muscle atonia (absence of muscle tone) and intermittent bursts of rapid eye movements, from which it gets its name. Muscle atonia in this state is interrupted by short bursts of phasic activity often accompanied by visible body jerks or twitches. The arousal threshold in REM sleep is variable.

These two sleep states are interrupted throughout the night by brief arousals characterised by EEG changes towards the wake state and an increase in muscle tone with accompanying movement. The arousals vary in duration from a few seconds to several minutes. The perception of these arousals by the individual depends on their duration and the time of night at which they occur (Knab and Engel, 1988).

Thus sleep is not a uniform state but is constantly changing throughout the night with intrusions by arousals resulting in body movements. In addition, visible jerks and movements may accompany K complexes and phasic increase in muscle tone in REM sleep.

Progression of sleep across the night

NREM and REM sleep alternate cyclically throughout the night. This cycling is present at birth, but the cycle time is 50–60 minutes in the newborn against 90 minutes in older children and adults (Carskadon and Dement, 1989). Although NREM and REM sleep are recognisable at birth, the development of adult-type NREM sleep with high-voltage synchronous slow waves requires a certain amount of brain maturity and emerges from 2–6 months of life (Carskadon and Dement, 1989). With consolidation of sleep during the night between 3 and 6 months of age (Coons, 1987), trends towards the adult pattern of distribution of NREM and REM sleep states through the night become apparent.

Sleep studies involving both young children and adults show that sleep is entered through NREM sleep. NREM sleep stages 3 and 4 dominate the sleep cycles in the early part of the night and the REM periods are short. As the night progresses, stages 1 and 2 of NREM sleep as well as REM sleep take up proportionately greater periods of each sleep cycle, so that morning awakening occurs from REM sleep or the light stages of NREM sleep. Stage 3 and 4 sleep are maximal in young children and decrease in favour of more stage 1 and 2 sleep with age. This explains why young children can be difficult to wake from the first sleep cycle. Both sleep states are interrupted by brief arousals, increasing in frequency and duration as the night progresses. Overall these occupy less than 5 per cent of the night (Carskadon and Dement, 1989).

Changes in other physiological parameters during sleep

Many physiological regulatory mechanisms are altered in sleep and vary in the two sleep states. These include respiration, blood flow, metabolic rate, thermoregulation and hormone production.

Respiration is not uniform in NREM stage 1 and 2 sleep, and shows regular waxing and waning (Bulow, 1963). Breathing is steady and regular in stages 3 and 4 of NREM sleep (Krieger *et al.*, 1983; Rist *et al.*, 1986). In REM sleep respiration is irregular with sudden change in respiratory amplitude and frequency associated with bursts of rapid eye movement which can be interrupted by central apnoeas lasting 10–30 seconds (Krieger, 1989).

There is a reduction in ventilatory response in sleep to hypoxia (low oxygen saturation in the blood) and hypercapnia (high carbon dioxide saturation in the blood). It is lower in NREM sleep than in wakefulness and lower in REM sleep than in NREM sleep (Douglas, 1989).

Basal metabolic rate generally falls during sleep. There is, however, an increase in metabolic rate in REM sleep in humans compared with NREM sleep (Glotzbach and Heller, 1989). There are parallel changes in other physiological parameters including a slight reduction in heart rate and a fall in blood pressure in NREM sleep, the lowest blood pressure measurements coinciding with stages 3 and 4 of sleep. Heart rate and systematic arterial blood pressure tend to be higher in REM sleep than in NREM sleep (Khatrie and Freis, 1967). However, heart rate and blood presure are very variable in REM sleep and are characterised by sudden increases which may even exceed the wake state at times.

Brain blood flow increases during sleep. The increase is slight in NREM sleep due to mild hypercapnia as a result of a decrease in minute ventilation (Santiago *et al.*, 1984). The increase can be more dramatic in REM sleep and is more than can be explained by hypercapnia alone. Alteration in autoregulation may be a possible contributory factor.

Thermoregulatory mechanisms remain intact in NREM sleep, although core temperature falls slightly. In contrast, temperature regulation is impaired during REM sleep and both shivering and thermal sweating are inhibited in this sleep stage (Glotzbach and Heller, 1989). Quality and quantity of sleep are also dependent on environmental temperature. Total sleep time is maximal in thermoneutrality ($31.5–33.5°C$) and decreases above and below environmental thermoneutrality (Glotzbach and Heller, 1989). There is a close interaction between the circadian body temperature rhythm and sleep/wake cycle. The circadian temperature rhythm is independent of environmental temperature. Sleep onset is most likely to occur near the nadir of body temperature and awakening during rise of body temperature (Czeisler *et al.*, 1980). It has also been suggested that decrease in core body temperature at sleep onset is essential for the evolution of deep sleep (Sewitch, 1987).

Several anterior pituitary hormones, the pineal hormone melatonin and cortisol are released in sinusoidal fashion over 24 hours, with this cycle being determined by several biological factors (see Parkes (1985a) for a review of hormonal changes in sleep). Two hormones whose release appears to have a direct link to the sleep/wake cycle are growth hormone and prolactin. Growth hormone release during sleep is dependent upon age. Below the age of three months sleep–related growth hormone peaks are not found. Growth hormone release is dependent on sleep onset from three months to puberty, with peak release occurring between NREM stages 3 and 4. This pattern of growth hormone secretion in relation to sleep continues in adult life.

Development and distribution of sleep patterns in human neonates and infants

Interest in infant sleep patterns has increased dramatically over the last twenty years. The study of the ontogeny of very early sleep patterns has become particularly important because the survival of increasingly premature babies has provided insight into some aspects of the development and maturation of the immature brain, reflected in the infants' regulation of their sleep/wake pattern.

Early studies in infants' sleep/wake patterns were based on observation of infant sleep behaviour during the day. Aserinsky and Kleitman (1955) first identified the quiet sleep (QS)/active sleep (AS) cycle in sleeping infants, the precursor of the NREM/REM cycle. This observational method of assessing sleep in babies was further developed by Prechtl and Beintema (1964) in term infants and then by Parmelee et al. (1972), who compared the sleep/wake state development of premature infants with full-term infants. Anders et al. (1985) elaborated on this method of assessing sleep/wake organisation in premature and full-term infants by analysis of all-night video somnograms of infants in their home environment.

Sleep in neonates and infants cannot be studied electrophysiologically using Rechtschaffen and Kales' criteria as, during this period of rapid brain maturation, there are various transitional sleep stages (which are indeterminate). In addition, a degree of cerebral maturity is required to produce a substrate for the occurrence of the high-voltage synchronous slow waves characteristic of non-REM sleep. However, Hoppenbrouwers et al. (1988) used polygraphs to study twenty normal-term infants at one week of age at monthly intervals up to four months of age, and again at six months of age. The physiological parameters used included EEG, eye movements, chin EMG, and ECG (electrocardiogram), as well as respiratory movements measured by impedance pneumography and measurement of expired gas and skin temperature. Their work has provided much needed electrophysiological normative data of the development and distribution of sleep in the first six months of life (see Hoppenbrouwers, 1987, p. 3).

Development of NREM/REM states in neonates

Neonates born before 30 weeks gestation spend 90 per cent of sleep time in REM sleep (active sleep) compared with 50 per cent at term. At 28 weeks gestation a tracé discontinua EEG pattern is identified, consisting of bursts of high-voltage irregular activity interrupted with periods of no activity for up to three minutes. This reflects the inability of the very immature brain to sustain continuous electrical activity. By 29 weeks gestation REM sleep can often be identified because of increased respiratory rate and increased eye movement (Smith, 1989).

Periods of quiet sleep are identified at around 32 weeks gestation (Sterman and Hoppenbrouwers, 1971). However, during this period of maturation, the distinction between NREM and REM is often difficult, so that some sleep is classed as indeterminate, making it a somewhat transitional period.

With progressive maturation there is a gradual increase in continuous electrical activity until term. At term, quiet sleep characterises the nature of NREM sleep; this sleep has a tracé alternant pattern of a 2–6 second burst of activity followed by 4–6 seconds of lower voltage in near absence of activity. At term the newborn spends two-thirds of a 24-hour period asleep, and by six months spends half the time asleep and half awake. The increase in wakefulness is at the cost of a reduction in REM sleep blocks, with the time spent in NREM sleep in a 24-hour period being remarkably stable (Coons, 1987). Sleep spindles develop at one month post-term as the tracé alternant pattern is replaced. K complexes appear by 5–6 months (Smith, 1989). As mentioned earlier, the high-voltage synchronous slow waves of stage 3 and 4 sleep emerge from 2 to 6 months of life (Carskadon and Dement, 1989).

After this there is a progressive increase towards the adult pattern, although the total sleep time and proportion of deep sleep will vary depending on age. There is also a progressive reduction in amplitude of the electrical activity in sleep until the post-pubertal period.

Development of sleep/wake cycle in neonates and infants

It has been established that a basic rest/activity cycle (BRAC) originates in foetal life (Sterman and Hoppenbrouwers, 1971) and is definable in the second half of gestation (Booth *et al.*, 1980; Parmelee *et al.*, 1967). There is controversy as to whether the fetus is ever truly awake. Animal studies suggest that the fetus is never awake but alternates between active sleep and quiet sleep. Movements such as swallowing, kicking and breathing occur in active sleep (Rigatto *et al.*, 1986).

Power spectra which are used to detect brain activity have shown a cycle time in the foetus between 40–60 minutes (Sterman and Hoppenbrouwers, 1971), which is similar to the sort of cycle length observed in pre-term infants at 36 weeks and term infants between one and six months of age (Stern *et al.*, 1973; Harper *et al.*, 1981).

Some of the seminal work in this area in infants was originally carried out by Parmelee and colleagues (1964). Their data were collected using behavioural observation by mothers throughout the day. This study followed children from birth to 16 weeks. They found that there was a relatively small decrease in the total hours of sleep per day over the 16 weeks, from 16.3 to 14.8 hours. However, the average daily continuous sleep period increased from 4 to 8.48 hours over 16 weeks and the average daily longest period of wakefulness increased from 2.39 to 3.56 hours. In the first week there were almost equal amounts of sleep during the day and night but by the sixteenth week infants slept double the amount of sleep at night as compared to the day. This favouring of sleep during the night was first evident during the second month of life and was better established by 3 to 4 months. From a clinical point of view, the most striking issue was the doubling in the longest sustained sleep period. The authors point out that these developments in sleep behaviour are part of a general maturation and learning process. Thus these changes correspond with other major behavioural changes in the infant during this time period. For example, the infant becomes free of primitive righting reflexes which dominate him as a newborn infant. He opens and closes his hands at will and follows people and objects freely with his eyes. He also smiles readily in social situations.

Before one month of age, the sleep/waking pattern is organised around 3–4 hourly feed times. Between 1 and 3 months of age, as the diurnal pattern begins to be established, it is influenced variably by environmental and maturational factors (Kleitman and Englemann, 1953). At around this time the redistribution of the sleep state takes place so that NREM sleep begins to dominate the beginning of the night and REM sleep later on (Hoppenbrouwers *et al.*, 1982). Around this 1 to 3 month period, the active sleep/quiet sleep cycle becomes remarkably regular. This excessive regularity of the alternating sleep states at this age may make the infant vulnerable because of an inability to respond to variations in the environment with the appropriate physiological response. This may have a role to play in increased susceptibility to sudden infant death syndrome (SIDS) around this age (Hoppenbrouwers, 1986).

Sleep states at 3 to 6 weeks of age are interrupted by frequent brief arousals. These are most frequent during REM sleep and probably represent 'pre-programmed' phasic self-stimulating brief arousals (Coons, 1987). Infants often wake from REM sleep when hypoxic or hypercapnic (McCulloch *et al.*, 1982; Ariagno *et al.*, 1980), suggesting that this sleep state is most sensitive to interruption in times of physiological necessity (Baker and McGinty, 1979). With cerebral maturation these arousals become less frequent. Anders *et al.* (1985) found the development of sleep continuity a useful predictor of mental function in premature infants. In particular, they found that mental performance at 24 weeks of age (as measured by the Bayley developmental scales) correlated with long quiet sleep periods early in the night. Furthermore, developmental quotients at 52 weeks were predicted by mature patterns of sustained sleep, namely infants who sleep for long periods and who sleep uninterrupted. In other words, there was a relationship in general between development and the maturity of the sleep/wake state organisation.

The same authors also noted that both preterm and term infants' ability to remain asleep continuously increases from four hours at two weeks to seven hours at one year. They found that, in general, the premature group have a tendency to more wakefulness at night at all ages in the first year, but this differed significantly from the term infant only at one year of age. They comment on the fact that most parents whose night is undisturbed think their child has slept longer. This is because some infants are able to soothe themselves back to sleep when they awake (quiet awakening), while others cry for parental attention and get labelled as 'night wakers.' Premature infants seem better self-soothers than term infants (Anders and Keener, 1985). The infants' sleep may of course be disturbed by discomfort such as snoring, colic (Weissbluth *et al.*, 1984) or excessive warmth (Wailoo *et al.*, 1990). Hunger may also be a cause in view of reports of breast-fed babies waking more frequently (Eaton-Evans and Dugdale, 1988).

Other physiological differences in the sleep of infants and older children

Periodic breathing in neonates alters between breathing intervals and apnoeas of 5–10 seconds' duration. In wake and quiet sleep it is regular. In REM sleep it is irregular (Rigatto, 1989; Prechtl, 1974). In addition, pulmonary reflexes, stretch receptors and irritant receptors are inactive during REM sleep, thus airway mechanisms for clearing are impaired in REM sleep (Phillipson, 1978; Hagan *et al.*, 1972). Respiration is further impaired in REM sleep by muscle atonia and intercostal muscle collapse, so that the work of the diaphragm is increased (Henderson-Smart and Read, 1979).

The changes in other physiological parameters, such as cerebral blood flow, heart rate, basal metabolic rate and thermoregulation, are similar to those seen in NREM and REM sleep states in older children and adults. However, the large proportion of sleep time spent in REM sleep by preterm and term neonates makes them vulnerable to the fluctuation in alteration in the physiological state in this period. Of particular importance is the disturbed thermoregulation in REM sleep, which has been implicated in sudden infant death syndrome (SIDS) as a result of increased heat production by overwrapping.

The circadian body temperature rhythm with a fall in night-time temperature similar to adults is established by 4 months of age (Lodemore *et al.*, 1991). This occurs in stages, between 4–8 weeks of age. The stabilisation of the temperature circadian rhythm coincides with longer nocturnal consolidation of sleep.

EEG and sleep patterns of infants as possible predictors of later intellectual development

We have already discussed the development of sleep continuity as a marker of cerebral maturation. Some authors have, however, studied specific EEG patterns of neonates and young infants as a way of assessing the maturation and integrity of a neurophysiological organisation. Most studies to date have concentrated on EEG patterns amongst clinical samples of infants, for example those with seizures, untreated hyperthyroidism or Down's syndrome. However, some recent studies have begun to look at EEG or state organisation and later development amongst infants without specific pathology at birth, and particularly those born prematurely (e.g. Ellingson et al., 1974; Thoman et al., 1980). Some studies find no relation between EEG or state organisation and later development among infants without specific pathology at birth (Ellingson et al., 1974; Tharp et al., 1981; Torres and Blaw, 1968). Other studies have found that some deviations in the expected state and EEG patterns were linked to later medical and/or behavioural difficulties (Crowell et al., 1982; Lombroso, 1982; Tharp et al., 1981; Thoman et al., 1976). A particularly interesting study has been carried out by Beckwith and Parmelee (1986). As part of a prospective longitudinal study of preterm infants, the sleep state organisation and EEG patterns were studied at term date in a group of preterm infants as an index of maturity and integrity of neurophysiological organisation that might have implications for their later development. Tracé alternant EEG patterns (as measured at 40 weeks conceptional age) were taken as the primary index of EEG and sleep maturity (see above). In general, children who at term date showed less tracé alternant pattern had lower IQs, beginning at four months and continuing to age 8. This, however, was not the case for children with low levels of tracé alternant patterns who were being reared in consistently attentive and responsive environments. By 24 months and continuing to age 8 they had IQs equal to those infants with more tracé alternant patterns. In general, it appears that the level of neurophysiological organisation as measured by the EEG at 40 weeks post conception in these premature infants was predictive of IQ at age 8. However, a stimulating, emotional environment was able to compensate amongst those who had more immature neurophysiological systems in the early months of life.

Beckwith and Parmelee's findings are potentially very important, in particular the apparent ability of infant EEG patterns to predict child development into the school-age period. However, these findings will need to be treated with caution until further research is done and replication studies carried out.

The function of sleep

In spite of 50 years of research the precise function of sleep remains controversial. A popular theory is that sleep is essential for either cerebral or body restitution. Workers that favour cerebral restitution as a major function of sleep have concentrated on REM sleep because of its association with dreaming (Dement and Kleitman, 1957). Jouvet (1975) suggested that REM sleep evolved to reprogramme innate behaviour in mammals who were at risk of losing it by advanced learned behaviour. Crick and Mitchison (1983), on the other hand, suggest that REM sleep is for 'unlearning' to avoid overloading of the neuronal network. It has also been argued that sleep plays an important role in memory but the evidence for this remains weak (Parkes 1985b).

Snyder (1966, 1969) suggested that sleep in mammals and birds was necessary to conserve energy to offset the cost of homeothermy. Continuing on this theme, Berger and Walker (1972) favoured the hypothesis that sleep reduced energy expenditure below that obtained by rest alone. They considered REM sleep as ectothermic and therefore as a vestige of the reptilian stage. However, the 10 to 15 per cent reduction in metabolic rate is not sufficient to explain the need for sleep.

Zepelin and Rechtschaffen's (1974) work elaborated on an alternative theory, that sleep with its enforced rest put a ceiling on energy expenditure, and that the diurnal organisation of the sleep/wake cycle prevents foraging at a time when it may be wasteful of energy and incur predatory danger (Meddis, 1977).

The cycle length of sleep appears to relate to the brain weight in different species and in individual species increases with maturation (Zepelin, 1989). On the other hand, the duration of daily sleep correlates with body weight. Linstedt and Boyce (1985) showed that, at thermoneutrality, survival time is a function of body size.[2] Thus small animals require more sleep to avoid exhausting their energy reserve. Horne (1988) believes that the restitution theory of sleep and the energy conservation theory are not mutually exclusive. He argues that sleep can be divided into core sleep and optional sleep. Core sleep occupies the first three sleep cycles and is represented predominantly by stages 3 and 4 of NREM sleep, and it is this sleep which is important for cerebral restitution. The remaining sleep he terms 'optional' sleep, which he considers to have an energy-conserving role in small animals or merely the function of occupying unproductive hours in other mammals. This sleep is represented by stage 2 NREM sleep.

Parmeggiani (1982) suggests that REM sleep is ontogenically primitive and is under rhombencephalic (brain stem and cerebellum) control, as opposed to the hypothalamic regulation of NREM sleep (ontogenically younger). Hence the amount of REM sleep in a species will correlate inversely with the degree of maturation of the hypothalamus. There is a view (Zepelin, 1989) that REM sleep in mature animals, though not a vestige of the reptilian stage, may be a carry over of foetal life where it has important functions in maintaining periods of activity in the developing foetus which is taken over by the wake state in the neonate. It is certainly difficult with the state of present knowledge to consider any physiologically useful function for this sleep which is characterised by a lack of themoregulation and by respiratory irregularities.

In summary, it can be said that the development of the sleep/wake cycle and the maturation of the different sleep states are closely linked to the integrity of the developing central nervous system. It has been suggested that the architecture and continuity of sleep may be a useful marker for the integrity of the developing brain, especially in the neonatal period, though further studies are needed.

There is no doubt, however, that an understanding of the development of the sleep/wake cycle, the maturation of different sleep stages with age, the progression of sleep through the night and the physiological changes accompanying sleep can enhance the understanding and management of clinical conditions frequently faced by paediatricians and other clinicians. These may range from the relatively benign, though sometimes socially devastating, problems of frequent nocturnal awakening by the infant and sleepwalking/night terrors in the toddler or older child, to more serious conditions related to cardio-respiratory instability or disturbance of thermal regulation, especially in the vulnerable group of infants such as the premature or the child compromised by another medical condition.

Notes

1. Spindles are an identifying feature of stage 2 sleep, consisting of spindle-shaped bursts of fast activity that last from 0.5 to 1.5 seconds. A K complex is a high-voltage sharp negative wave, followed by a positive wave lasting more than 0.5 seconds and occurring in stage 2 sleep. They occur spontaneously, in response to external stimuli or in response to changes in the activity of the internal autonomic system.
2. Thermoneutrality is the range of environmental temperature when core temperature can be maintained without an increase in metabolic rate.

References

Anders, T.F. and Keener, M.A. (1985), 'Developmental course of night time sleep–wake patterns in full-term and premature infants during the first year of life. I', *Sleep*, 8, pp. 173–92.

Anders, T.F., Keener, M.A. and Kraemer, H. (1985), 'Sleep–wake state organisation, neonatal assessment and development in premature infants during the first year of life. II', *Sleep*, 8, pp. 193–206.

Ariagno, R., Nagel, L. and Guilleminault, C. (1980), 'Waking and ventilatory responses in near miss SIDS infants during sleep', *Sleep*, 3, pp. 351–9.

Aserinsky, E. and Kleitman, N. (1955), 'A motility cycle in sleeping infants as manifested by ocular and gross bodily activity', *Journal of Applied Physiology*, 8, pp. 11–13.

Baker, T.L. and McGinty, D.J. (1979), 'Sleep–waking patterns in hypoxic kittens', *Developmental Psychobiology*, 12, pp. 561–75.

Beckwith, L. and Parmelee, A.H. Jr (1986), 'EEG patterns of preterm infants, home environment and later IQ', *Child Development*, 57, pp. 777–89.

Berger, R.J. and Walker, J.M. (1972), 'A polygraphic study of sleep in the tree shrew

(Tupais glis)', *Brain Behaviour Evolution*, 5, pp. 54–69.

Booth, C.L., Leonard, H.L. and Thomas, E.B. (1980), 'Sleep states and behaviour patterns in preterm and full term infants', *Neuropaediatrics*, 11, p. 354.

Bulow, K. (1963), 'Respiration and wakefulness in man', *Acta Physiologica Scandinavica*, 5, pp. 1–110.

Carskadon, M.A. and Dement, W.C. (1989), 'Normal human sleep: an overview', in H. Kryger, T. Roth, W.C. Dement (eds), *Principles and Practice of Sleep Medicine* (Philadelphia, PA: W.B. Saunders), pp. 3–13.

Coons, S. (1987), 'Development of sleep and wakefulness during the first 6 months of life', in C. Guilleminault (ed.), *Sleep and its Disorder in Children* (New York: Raven), pp. 17–27.

Crick, F. and Mitchison, G. (1983), 'The function of dream sleep', *Nature*, 304, pp. 111–13.

Crowell, D.H., Kapuniai, L.E., Boychut, R.B., Light, M.J. and Hodgman, J.E. (1982), 'Daytime sleep state organisation in three month old infants', *Electroencephalography and Clinical Neurophysiology*, 53, pp. 36–47.

Czeisler, C.A., Weitzman, E.D., Moors-Ede, M.C., Zimmerman, J.C. and Knaver, R.S. (1980), 'Human sleep. Its duration and organisation depend on circadian phase', *Science*, 210, pp. 1264–7.

Dement, W.C. and Kleitman, M. (1957), 'The relations of eye movements during sleep to dream activity; an objective method for the study of dreaming', *Journal of Experimental Psychology*, 53, pp. 339–46.

Douglas, N.J. (1989), 'Control of ventilation during sleep', in M.H. Kryger, T. Roth and W.C. Dement (eds), *Principles and Practice of Sleep Medicine* (Philadelphia, PA: W.B. Saunders), pp. 249–56.

Eaton-Evans, J. and Dugdale, A.E. (1988), 'Sleep patterns of infants in the first year of life', *Archives of Disease in Childhood*, 63, pp. 647–9.

Ellingson, R.J., Dutch, S.J. and McIntire, M.S. (1974), 'EEGs of prematures: 3–8 year follow up study', *Developmental Psychobiology*, 7, pp. 529–38.

Glotzbach, S.F. and Heller, H. (1989), 'Thermo regulation', in H. Kryger, T. Roth and W.C. Dement (eds), *Principles and Practice of Sleep Medicine* (Philadelphia, PA: W.B. Saunders), pp. 300–9.

Hagan, R.A.C., Bryan, C.A., Bryan, M.H. and Gulston, G. (1972), 'The effect of sleep state on interostal muscle activity and rib cage motion', *Physiologist*, 19, p. 214.

Harper, R.M., Leake, B., Miyahara. L., Hoppenbrouwers, T., Sterman, M.B. and Hodgman, J.E. (1981), 'Development of ultradian periodicity and coalescence at 1 cycle per hour in electroencephalographic activity', *Experimental Neurology*, 73, pp. 127–43.

Henderson-Smart, D.J. and Read, D.J.C. (1979), 'Reduced lung volume during behavioural active sleep in the newborn', *Journal of Applied Physiology*, 46, pp. 1081–5.

Hoppenbrouwers, T. (1986), 'Ontogenesis of sleep and waking', in M.B. Sterman, J.E. Hodgman, C.R. Stark and H.J. Hoffman (eds), *Ontogeny of Sleep and Cardiopulmonary Regulation: Factors related to risk for sudden infant death syndrome* (Washington, DC: NICHD).

Hoppenbrouwers, T. (1987), 'Sleep in infants', in C. Guilleminault (ed.), *Sleep and its Disorders in Children* (New York: Raven).

Hoppenbrouwers, T., Hodgman, J.E., Arawaka, K., Geidel, S.A. and Sterman, M.B. (1988), 'Sleep and waking states in infancy: normative studies', *Sleep*, 11, pp. 387–402.

Hoppenbrouwers, T., Hodgman, J.E., Harper, R.M. and Sterman, M.B. (1982),

'Temporal distribution of sleep states, somatic activity and autonomic activity during the first half year of life', *Sleep*, 5, pp. 131–44.

Horne, J. (1988), 'Why do we sleep?', in J. Horne (ed.), *The Functions of Sleep in Humans and Other Mammals* (Oxford: Oxford University Press), pp. 310–14.

Jones, B.E. (1989), 'Basic mechanisms of sleep–wake states', in H. Kryger, T. Roth and W.C. Dement (eds), *Principles and Practice of Sleep Medicine* (Philadelphia, PA: W.B. Saunders), pp. 121–38.

Jouvet, M. (1975), 'The function of dreaming: a neurophysiologist's point of view', in M.S. Gazzaniga and C. Blakemore (eds), *Handbook of Psychobiology* (New York: Academic), pp. 499–527.

Khatrie, I.M. and Freis, E.D. (1967), 'Haemodynamic changes during sleep', *Journal of Applied Physiology*, 22, pp. 867–73.

Kleitman, N. and Camille, W. (1932), 'Studies on the physiology of sleep VI. The behavior of decorticated dogs', *American Journal of Physiology*, 100, p. 474.

Kleitman, N. and Englemann, T.G. (1953), 'Sleep characteristics in infants', *Journal of Applied Physiology*, 6, p. 269–82.

Knab, B. and Engel, R.R. (1988), 'Perception of waking and sleeping: possible implications for the evaluation of insomnia', *Sleep*, 11, pp. 265–72.

Krieger, J. (1989), 'Breathing during sleep in normal subjects', in M.H. Kryger, T. Roth and W.C. Dement (eds), *Principles and Practice of Sleep Medicine* (Philadelphia, PA: W.B. Saunders), pp. 257–68.

Krieger, J., Turlot, J.C., Mangin, P. and Kurtz, D. (1983), 'Breathing during sleep in normal young and elderly subjects: hypopneas, apneas and correlated factors', *Sleep*, 6, pp. 108–20.

Lindstedt, S.L. and Boyce, M.S. (1985), 'Seasonality, fasting endurance and body size in mammals', *American Naturalist*, 125, pp. 873–8.

Lodemore, M., Peterson, S.A. and Wailoo, M.P. (1991), 'Development of night time temperature rhythm over the first 6 months of life', *Archives of Disease in Childhood*, 66, pp. 521–4.

Lombroso, C.T. (1982), 'Some aspects of EEG polygraphy in newborns at risk for neurological disorders', in P.A. Buser, W.C. Cobb and T. Okuma (eds), *Kyoto Symposia (EEG Supplement No. 36)* (Amsterdam: Elsevier), pp. 652–63.

McCulloch, K., Brouillette, R.T., Guzetta, A.J. and Hunt, C.E. (1982), 'Arousal responses in near miss sudden infant death syndrome and in normal infants', *Journal of Pediatrics*, 101, pp. 911–17.

Meddis, R. (1977), *The Sleep Instinct* (London: Routledge and Kegan Paul).

Moruzzi, G. (1972), 'The sleep waking cycle', *Egreb. Physiol*, 64, p. 1.

Moruzzi, G. and Magoun, H.W. (1949), 'Brain stem reticular formation and activation of the EEG', *Electroencephalography and Clinical Neurophysiology*, 1, p. 455.

Parkes, J.D. (1985a), 'Circadian rhythms and sleep', in J.D. Parkes (ed.), *Sleep and Its Disorders* (London: W.B. Saunders), pp. 121–83.

Parkes, J.D. (1985b), 'Normal sleep, its variants and related states', in J.D. Parkes (ed.), *Sleep and Its Disorders* (London: W.B. Saunders), pp. 5–70.

Parmeggiani, P.L. (1982), 'Regulation of physiological functions during sleep in mammals', *Experientia*, 38, pp. 1405–8.

Parmelee, A.H., Stern, E. and Harris, M. (1972), 'Maturation of respiration in prematures and young infants', *Neuropaediatrics*, 3, pp. 294–304.

Parmelee, A.H., Wenner, W.H., Akiyama, Y., Schultz, M. and Stern, E. (1967), 'Sleep states in premature infants', *Developmental Medicine and Child Neurology*, 9, p. 70.

Parmelee, A.H. Jr., Wenner, W.H. and Schulz, H.R. (1964), 'Infant sleep patterns: from birth to 16 weeks of age', *Journal of Pediatrics*, 65, pp. 576–82.

Phillipson, E.A. (1978), 'Control of breathing during sleep', *American Review of Respiratory Disorders*, 118, pp. 909–39.

Prechtl, H. (1974), 'The behavioural states of the newborn infant (a review)', *Brain Research*, 76, p. 185.

Prechtl, H.F.R. and Beintema, D. (1964), 'The neurological examination of the full term newborn infant', in *Clinics in Developmental Medicine 12* (London: Spastics Society and Heinemann).

Rechtschaffen, A. and Kales, A. (eds) (1968), *A Manual of Standardised Terminology, Techniques and Scoring System for Sleep Stages of Human Subjects* (Los Angeles: UCLA Brain Information Service/Brain Research Institute).

Rigatto, H. (1989), 'Control of breathing during sleep in the fetus and neonate', in H. Kryger, T. Roth and W.C. Dement (eds), *Principles and Practice of Sleep Medicine* (Philadelphia, PA: W.B. Saunders), pp. 237–48.

Rigatto, H., Moore, M. and Cates, D. (1986), 'Fetal breathing and behaviour measured through a double wall plexiglas window in sleep', *Journal of Applied Physiology*, 61, p. 160.

Rist, K.E., Daubenspeck, J.A. and McGovern, J.F. (1986), 'Effects of non REM sleep upon respiratory drive and the respiratory pump in humans', *Respiratory Physiology*, 63, pp. 241–56.

Santiago, T.V., Guerra, E., Neubauer, J.A. and Edelman, N.H. (1984), 'Correlation between ventilation and brain blood flow during sleep', *Journal of Clinical Investigation*, 73, pp. 497–506.

Sewitch, D.E. (1987), 'Slow wave sleep deficiency insomnia: a problem in thermo downregulation of sleep onset', *Psychophysiology*, 24, pp. 200–15.

Smith, S. (1989), 'Sleep disorders in children', in C.V. Swaiman (ed.), *Pediatric Neurology Vol. 1* (Toronto: Mosby), pp. 149–56.

Snyder, F. (1966), 'Towards an evolutionary theory of dreaming', *American Journal of Psychiatry*, 123, pp. 121–36.

Snyder, F. (1969), 'Sleep and REM as biological enigmas', in A. Kales (ed.), *Sleep: Physiology and pathology* (Philadelphia, PA: J.B. Lippincott), pp. 266–80.

Sterman, M.B. and Hoppenbrouwers, T. (1971), 'The development of sleep–waking and rest–activity patterns from fetus to adult in man', in M.B. Sterman, D.J. McGinty and A.M. Adinolfi (eds), *Brain Development and Behavior* (New York: Academic), pp. 203–27.

Stern, E.L., Parmelee, A.H. and Harris, M.A. (1973), 'Sleep state periodicity in prematures and young infants', *Developmental Psychobiology*, 6, pp. 357–65.

Tharp, B.R., Cukier, F. and Monod, N. (1981), 'The prognostic value of the electroencephalogram in premature infants', *Electroencephalography and Clinical Neurophysiology*, 5, pp. 219–36.

Thoman, E.G., Denenberg, V.H., Sievel, J., Zeidner, L. and Becker, P. (1980), 'Behavioural state profiles in infancy are predictive of late medical or behavioural dysfunction', *Neuropaediatrics*, 12, pp. 45–54.

Thoman, E.G., Korner, A.F. and Kraemer, H.C. (1976), 'Individual consistency in behavioural states in neonates', *Developmental Psychobiology*, 9, pp. 271–83.

Torres, F. and Blaw, M.E. (1968), 'Longitudinal EEG – clinical correlations in children from birth to 4 years of age', *Pediatrics*, **41**, pp. 945–54.

Wailoo, M.P., Peterson, S.A. and Whittaker, H. (1990), 'Disturbed nights and 3–4 month old infants: the effects of feeding and thermal environment', *Archives of Disease in Childhood*, **65**, 499–501.

Weissbluth, M., Davies, A.J. and Poacher, J. (1984), 'Night waking in 4–8 month old infants', *Journal of Paediatrics*, **104**, pp. 477–80.

Zepelin, H. (1989), 'Mammalian sleep', in H. Kryger, T. Roth and W.C. Dement (eds), *Principles and Practice of Sleep Medicine* (Philadelphia, PA: W.B. Saunders), pp. 30–49.

Zepelin, H. and Rechtschaffen, A. (1974), 'Mammalian sleep, longevity and energy metabolism', *Brain Behaviour and Evolution*, **10**, pp. 425–70.

Chapter 8

The development of sleeping difficulties

David Messer, *University of Hertfordshire, and*
Martin Richards, *University of Cambridge*

Amantum Irae

In going to my naked bed as one that would
    have slept,
I heard a wife sing to her child, that long before
    had wept;
She sighed sore and sang full sweet, to bring the
    babe to rest,
That would not cease but cried still, in sucking
    at her breast.
She was full weary of her watch, and grieved
    with her child,
She rocked it and rated it, till that on her it
    smiled.
Then did she say, Now I have found this proverb
    true to prove,
The falling out of faithful friends renewing is of
    love.

She said that neither king nor prince nor lord
    could live aright.
Until their puissance they did prove, their
    manhood and their might.
When manhood can be matched so that fear can
    take no place,
Then weary works make warriors each other to
    embrace,
And left their force that failed them, which did
    consume the rout,
That might before have lived their time, their
    strength and nature out;
Then did she sing as one that thought no man
    could her reprove,
The falling out of faithful friends renewing is of
    love.

Richard Edwards (1523–66)

Introduction

About a quarter of all infants are still waking regularly at night – or at least waking their parents – at the end of the first year of their lives. Most parents find this a very disruptive and depressing pattern of behaviour and it frequently leads them to seek professional advice or to turn to a self-help book or friends for help. These sources present a wide spectrum of views and strategies. It seems that little of this is of much help, judging by the continuing high prevalence and persistence of the problem.

Night waking has also provoked much research, but here too we find a diversity of evidence and little sign of a clear and consistent picture of why some families suffer from this problem. Perhaps a major cause of this inconsistency is that we are dealing with a complex problem or, indeed, a complex set of problems, which are not clearly defined. Thus research studies may not always be addressing the same issues. So we need to begin with some definitions to obtain a clear picture of the phenomena under discussion.

Our scope will be limited to the preschool years and we will devote most of our attention to infancy, which will be somewhat arbitrarily defined as the first two years of life. During the first two years the total sleep time for infants gradually declines and a clear day/night cycle of sleeping is established. A majority of children (and here we are drawing our data from the industrialised world), continue to have a daytime nap into their second year, but this is generally quite brief – an hour or so – and most sleep takes place at night. Studies based on direct recording of infants' sleep, either by EEG or time-lapse video, show that a night's sleep for an infant is in fact broken up into a number of sequences of sleep states which are interspersed by waking periods. These waking periods average five per night at two months declining to one and a half per night at nine months (Anders, 1978). Parents' awareness of their child's waking is likely to depend on whether or not the child cries during these waking periods, where the child sleeps in relation to the parent, and how often parents check to see if the infant is asleep.

It will be clear that there could be a considerable difference between measures of night waking derived from physiological recording or filming and those which are based on parental reports. In the latter case, parents can only record waking that they are aware of and this will usually mean waking periods when the infant cries. The relative position of parents, other siblings and the babies is also likely to be of importance. Infants that sleep in the same room or bed as the parents are more likely to have their waking periods noted. Thus parental measures of night waking will contain an element of parental behaviour and many families will only record wake periods when the baby cries. However, it is important to bear in mind that different methods of data collection allow investigators to answer different questions about children's sleeping. Parental reports of night waking and their feelings about this are appropriate measures for investigations which are concerned with the effect of night waking on parents. In contrast, other methods of data collection which can give a direct measure of night waking are appropriate for investigations of changes in sleep patterns during development, in relation to factors like neurological development or patterns of caregiving.

Whether or not night waking is regarded as a problem by parents, or indeed researchers, will depend on what they believe to be normal. Parents may also differ in their tolerance of night waking. Very few parents believe that infants below the age of three to four months will sleep through the night without interruption. Therefore, night waking is seldom seen as a problem before this age. If there are complaints about a young baby's evening or night-time activity, it is usually about crying rather than waking. It may be that babies reported as crying excessively in the early months will at a later age be seen as having problems with sleeping (Bernal, 1972). Thus, there may be considerable overlap between crying problems on one hand and night waking on the other.

There is a further issue here: even though parents of young infants regard frequent waking as normal and do not see it as a problem, it is still possible that such behaviour affects their feelings and behaviour. Another point that needs to be made is that, even after four months, not all babies waking regularly at night are regarded as having a night waking problem. In a recent postal survey of one year olds, mothers were asked how many nights per week their babies woke and whether or not they thought there was a night waking problem (Scott and Richards, 1989). While 10 per cent of those whose babies woke on five or more nights a week did not regard this as a difficulty, 37 per cent of those whose babies woke less often than this reported there being a problem. Night waking is not the only sleeping problem that parents report. There may also be problems in getting infants off to sleep or with early waking. This survey found that these other problems are less frequent. There tends to be an association between the three kinds of problem and 4 per cent of infants were recorded as having difficulties in all three areas.

In summary, it is important to separate a number of related, but distinct, concepts of night waking, each of which will have its own aetiology and associations with other factors. Unless this is done we suggest that the field will remain confused. As far as night waking is concerned, we suggest that there are four principal concepts which are related to the method of measurement. (A similar list could be made for other aspects of sleep-wake behaviour.)

1. Night waking as assessed by physiological (EEG) means or direct observation of an infant.
2. Patterns of sleeping and waking by parental report.
3. Night waking problems as reported by parents.
4. Night waking problems as defined by a researcher on the basis of one or more of the above.

To add confusion to an already complex picture, not only are there different conceptual approaches in studying children's sleeping but different sampling procedures are associated with them. Some studies collect information about children who have been referred to health professionals because of the children's sleeping difficulty, while other studies select their samples on some normative basis (this can range from attempts to obtain representative samples, to ones which only contain healthy infants). With the former method of sampling, studies often compare the referred children with a control group, and in some cases the referred children may undergo treatment. With the latter method of sampling, the studies are often longitudinal and comparisons are usually made between a group which has high levels of night waking with the rest of the sample to discover if differences exist between them. Thus, although there is likely to be an overlap in the characteristics of families who have been referred and those that have high levels of night waking, it is uncertain how high an overlap this is, and as a result there may be differences in the findings according to the sampling method employed.

Another difference between studies is in the way that night-time is defined. As Bernal (1973) points out, there is considerable ambiguity about how the term night waking can be used when one takes into account seasonal variations and differences between parents in the way they use the term. Furthermore, experimenter definitions also vary, with the start of night being considered to occur anytime between 6.00 pm and midnight, and the end of night between 5 and 8 am.

In reviewing the literature on the development of sleeping difficulties and night waking we will first consider longitudinal normative studies of night waking which have either employed parental reports or have employed other methods of observation. The second section consists of a review of the factors which have been investigated for a possible association with sleeping difficulties. The implications of these findings are considered in an overview, where we propose a model of the aetiology of sleeping difficulties.

Longitudinal studies of children's sleeping

Prospective longitudinal studies of sleeping patterns supply information about the amount of night waking, and either indirectly or directly the prevalence of sleeping difficulties. Studies are presented according to the age range which has been investigated. In general these studies concern the amount and type of sleep disturbance rather than whether or not it is seen as a problem.

Parental reports about children's sleeping

A much quoted American study of early sleep patterns was conducted by Parmelee *et al.* (1964) who used a sleep chart filled in by largely middle-class mothers to obtain a longitudinal record of sleeping between birth and 22 weeks (see Zaiwalla and Stein, chapter 7). The longest period of sleep per 24 hours recorded by the mother was 4.1 hours in the first week, 4.6 in the fourth, 6.5 in the eighth, 7.7 in the twelfth, and 8.5 in the sixteenth. The authors comment that this was the most dramatic change observed in their study. Parmelee *et al.* regard these changes as part of the maturation of infants' neurological functioning, though they provided no evidence to support this speculation.

Moore and Ucko (1957), in one of the first large-scale longitudinal studies, collected data about sleep in the first year (3 to 52 weeks) from 205 English families. The information was obtained by various means: by interviews at a Study Centre, by parents keeping daily records, and by home interviews. Two measures were obtained: the age at which infants had slept through the night at least six nights per week for four weeks, and the 'rough estimate' of the number of nights when the baby woke in a year.

Moore and Ucko (1957), using a subsample of 104 cases, found that by three months 70 per cent of the babies had ceased to be reported to wake in the night, by four months 81 per cent had achieved this, and by ten months 91 per cent had achieved this (i.e. 9 per cent never settled throughout the year). The figures suggest that most children will be sleeping through the night by three to four months. In the first year there was a weak significant relationship between sleep patterns at younger and older ages ($r = 0.21$). Nearly half the sample were described as suffering from a relapse in night waking (this was not defined), with most children showing a relapse between seven and nine months.

Bernal (1973) has published data about night waking (defined as regular waking at fourteen months by maternal report) from the Cambridge Longitudinal Study (Richards and Bernal, 1972). 24 of 77 infants were waking regularly at 14 months. Parental diaries showed that the problem group (defined at 14 months) were more wakeful and irritable during the first 10 days of life. At 8, 14, 20 and 30 weeks the problem group showed a continuing pattern of shorter sleep bouts at night.

Jacklin *et al.* (1980) used parent diaries from a single day to examine sleeping at 6, 12, 18, 26 and 33 months in American children. Their sample at each age varied between 63 and 145 reports. They found that the total time asleep for a 24-hour period remained stable between 6 and 12 months, then decreased from 13.8 hours at 12 months to 11.3 hours at 33 months. The longest period of sleep increased steadily between 6 and 18 months (9.0 to 10.0 hours) and then remained stable between 18 and 33 months. The number of sleep/wake transitions decreased steadily from 8.5 at 6 months to 4.1 at 33 months. Total sleep and longest period of sleep showed significant correlations of around 0.4 between most of the adjacent age points. The longest period of wakefulness was not stable between age points, nor was the number of sleep/wake transitions. Interestingly, a retest on the measures for a subsample gave correlations between 0.20 and 0.90, with most being in between 0.50 and 0.70. In addition, 90 per cent agreement was found between data derived from these diaries and time-lapse video.

A picture of sleeping in the preschool years is provided by Beltramini and Hertzig (1983), who used detailed longitudinal interviews with mothers to examine sleeping at 1, 2, 3, 4 and 5 years of age (the children were first seen in 1956 as part of a longitudinal study). The proportion of children who exhibited night waking at least once a week showed a small increase across the age range: there was an increase from 57 per cent at 1 year to 66 per cent in the third year, and thereafter a modest decline to 61 per cent at 5 years, but these changes were not statistically significant. A substantial proportion of the children woke at least every night and this did not change significantly with age (highest 33 per cent at 3 years, lowest 19 per cent at 5 years). Anxiety and fears at night increased with age, there being substantially more nightmares reported at 3, 4 and 5 years (28, 39 and 38 per cent, respectively) than at 1 and 2 years (5 and 9 per cent). In addition, requests for treasured objects were significantly higher at 2, 3 and 4 years (46, 50 and 42 per cent, respectively) than at 1 and 5 years (18 and 20 per cent). With increasing age, bedtime became more problematic and took longer. There was a steady increase up to 4 years in the number of children who required a bedtime routine of more than 30 minutes (6 per cent at 1 year, 30 per cent at 4 years and 23 per cent at 5 years), and who needed more than 30 minutes to fall asleep (26 per cent at 1 year, 69 per cent at 4 years and 66 per cent at 5 years); all measures showed significant overall age differences. There was a significant increase across the whole range in the number of children who when put to bed recalled their parents at least once (14 per cent at 1 year, 50 per cent at 5 years).

In contrast to the previous studies, which suggest a degree of stability in children's sleeping, Van Tassel (1985) failed to find a relationship between sleep difficulties at different ages. However, her study collected data across a wide range of ages (15 to 27 months) and retested the children 9–12 months later, some in a laboratory and some by postal questionnaire. Thus, lack of standardisation may partly account for this failure.

Other methods of collecting data on children's sleep

Various methods, beside parental report, have been employed to collect information about children's sleeping. The recording methods range from time-lapse infrared video to EEG recordings, activity recordings and recordings of heart rate and respiration. Unfortunately, most studies have been made on infants who are less than six months old. In some of these studies the recordings are made at home, in others recordings have been made in a laboratory. With increasing age one would expect the latter situation to produce findings of less validity. One difference between these studies and those using parental reports is that they have tended to investigate a sample of infants selected according to some criteria, i.e. all have uncomplicated deliveries or all are low-birth-weight infants.

Coons and Guilleminault (1982) examined EEG activity in the first 6 months of life in 31 infants (see chapter 7). The recordings took place in a hospital with sleep states being scored in 30 second epochs as outlined by Anders *et al.* (1971) and were derived from EEG recordings at 3, 4, 5 and 6 months. The findings are broadly similar to Parmelee *et al.*'s: by 3 months sleep was found to occur more at night than day. Over the first 6 months there was a gradual decline in the total time spent asleep (905 minutes at 3 weeks, 733 minutes at 6 months). No significant differences were found between the previous nights' sleep at home as assessed by using a video recorder and the EEG data used in this study.

Hoppenbrouwers *et al.* (1988) studied 20 healthy infants from 1 week to 6 months using polygraph records in a laboratory. Reduction in variability occurred at 3–4 months but the authors suggest that the variability among and within infants casts doubt on the usefulness of polygraph records for identifying abnormalities. Siminoff and Stores (1987) refer to unpublished material which shows that parents' sleep diaries correspond to polygraph records. However, Anders and Sostek (1976) criticise polygraph studies conducted in laboratories for having a first-night effect which reduces the amount of active REM sleep.

Video recordings of sleep during the first year have been obtained by Anders and Keener (1985). The sample consisted of 40 full term and 24 premature infants (matched on conceptual age) who were regularly observed by time-lapse video somnography between 2 and 52 weeks of age in their home. The video recordings were conducted on a ratio of 1 hour of recording to 18 hours of observation. Using this data source, infants' sleep was categorised into 4 states (quiet sleep, active sleep, awake, out of crib). Changes in the proportion of quiet sleep and active sleep were not large over the first year. The authors comment on an interesting finding that, even at 1 year, infants typically sleep for 6–7 hours at night, then there is a brief period of awakening, which is followed by more sleep.

Thoman and Whitney (1989) used an activity monitor to record the sleeping of 20 healthy infants one day each week for the first 5 weeks of life. In contrast to previous studies, which had difficulty in identifying stable features of early sleeping (other than total time asleep) they were able to report stable individual differences in quiet sleep, active/quiet transitional sleep, active sleep, sleep/wake transitions, and waking. They also replicated a previous study (Thoman and Glazier, 1987) which found high levels of agreement between a computer analysis of activity levels during sleep and systematic observations of behaviour by trained personnel (mean agreement 86 per cent, range 76–98 per cent).

Summary

Parental reports about sleep patterns indicate that, from about 3–4 months of age, most infants are thought to sleep through the night. However, a substantial proportion of children, between a third to a fifth, will continue to be recorded as waking regularly through the preschool years, and this and related problems have a high probability of continuing. As the children become older, problems in settling at night become more pronounced. Studies which have employed time-lapse video indicate that, even after 3–4 months of age, children wake up briefly during the night, and this is not detected by parents. The number of such wakenings appear to diminish with increasing age but, as yet, we have no information about when and if such awakenings no longer occur.

The findings from automatic recordings or time-lapse recordings should not be accepted uncritically. These methods of recording do not produce perfect agreement when attempts have been made to check their reliability, and they may be subject to various types of error. Some awakenings may be missed when using time-lapse recordings. Furthermore, there is the question of how night waking should be defined with automatic recordings, and whether brief periods of waking should be included in such a definition.

Factors associated with sleeping difficulties

Views about the aetiology of sleeping difficulties

Before going on to consider the factors associated with sleeping difficulties, it is worth identifying different viewpoints about the aetiology of this condition. The main controversy about sleeping difficulties has been whether they are products of child characteristics or of parental behaviour, or both. It is easy to characterise authors as having opposing views, but opinions are often more subtle than this, with an awareness of the interacting influences of infant and parent on one another. Furthermore, despite the relatively high number of studies, there are surprisingly few detailed discussions of the aetiology of this condition. This may in part be because the studies have usually involved correlations, so that it is difficult to separate out the influence of the child on the parent, and *vice versa*.

The earliest studies of sleeping have tended to adopt the view that infant characteristics determine sleeping patterns. For example, Moore and Ucko (1957) suggest that the attainment of sleeping through the night is the result of a 'biological adaptation, [that] requires no consciously directed training by the parents' (p. 341), and propose that if sleeping is not established by four to five months then adjustment may be difficult because a type of sensitive period is passed. However, the authors also go on to comment that some types of parental behaviour are associated with sleeping difficulties and, as a result, it is difficult to disentangle parental influence from the influence of the baby on the parent. They also raise the possibility of sleeping difficulties being a product of the mismatch between parental and child characteristics.

Another view has been that sleeping difficulties are associated with complications or difficulties at the birth of the child. Blurton Jones *et al.* (1978) argue that their data support the view that obstetric factors and associated high levels of activity in infancy are the best predictors of later sleeping problems.

Bernal (1973) also has findings which implicate events during pregnancy and labour with sleeping difficulties. Bernal (1973) observed that 'the course of delivery is associated with greater irritability and wakefulness of the babies in the [sleeping] problem group' (p. 766). However, she also points out that the relation was not an absolute one, there being entries in all the cells of her cross-classification of sleeping difficulties and events at birth. Extrapolating from these findings, Bernal speculates that there may be a relation of sleeping problems with factors earlier in the pregnancy. She suggests that the sleeping problem group may have mothers who in the first ten days are more responsive to their infants. This leads her to suggest that infants who are irritable and have a responsive mother will later have sleeping difficulties (see also Blurton Jones *et al.* (1978)). We develop an interactive model of this kind later in the chapter. The theme of infant irritability being associated with sleeping difficulties has also been taken up by Carey (1974), who claims that sleep problem babies have a lower sensory threshold at six months.

Parental management of infants has also been discussed as a cause of sleeping difficulties. Zuckerman *et al.* (1987) suggest that 'persistent sleeping problems are part of more pervasive behavioral difficulties between parent and child involving limits and boundaries'. Adherents of the behavioural management approach to treatment maintain that, even if parental behaviour was not instrumental in causing the sleeping difficulties, it is responsible for maintaining them. This is explicitly acknowledged by Douglas and Richman (1982), while Seymour *et al.* (1983) argue that the success of behavioural management programmes suggests that parental behaviour maintains children's night waking. In a similar vein, Van Tassel (1985) states 'there is strong evidence to indicate that sleeping practices, specifically those that interfere with continuous night-time sleep, are strong predictors of sleeping disturbance in both early and late infancy'. Her data reveals a relation between night feeds, crying before falling asleep, sleeping in parents' bed, going to the parents' bed on awakening and sleeping difficulties.

Another feature of parental behaviour which is seen as a possible influence on sleeping patterns is breast-feeding and weaning. Carey (1975) has speculated that breast-feeding may set up expectations in infants that they are more likely to be picked up and fed when they fuss. Elias *et al.* (1986) have argued that breast-feeding and a later age of weaning are associated with night waking, while the work of Lozoff *et al.* (1984) suggests that there may be a complex interplay between sleeping difficulties, breast-feeding, weaning and co-sleeping.

The psychoanalytic perspective has been used to explain why sleeping difficulties are often associated with anxiety, stressful life events and maternal depression both before and after the birth of the child (Daws, 1985). Guedeney and Kreisler (1987) suggest that there is an association 'between a very active, excited child, a mother–child relationship characterized by hyperstimulation, a mother with many phobic concerns about the child, and subsequent sleep disorders'. Thus, sleeping difficulties are seen as part of a wider set of problems between the mother and infant, though there remains a need to quantify these relations.

In reviewing the literature on the causes of sleeping difficulties we will organise the material to reflect our model of the influences on this behaviour. It is important to note that our model is neither biological or social, nor is it assumed that night waking is caused by either the mother or the baby. We suggest that congenital characteristics predispose infants to later sleeping problems. Such infants may well be more responsive to stimuli, more difficult to entrain to a diurnal rhythm, and have more difficulty in soothing themselves. Here we should note that, to avoid misunderstanding, we use the term 'congenital' to describe differences that are apparent in fetal life without intending any implication about the developmental processes that may have created such differences.

We also assume that parental care practices (usually of the mother) will influence the development of infants' sleeping patterns. These practices are in turn influenced, not only by characteristics of the infant, but also be cultural expectations, maternal attitudes, experiences of labour, maternal stress and the social and physical organisation of the household. Our concept of sleeping difficulties is a relational one and we see the problem residing in the relationship between mother (or parent) and child. For the mother (and the infant) there may be different paths that lead to sleeping difficulties, for example some parents may be disposed to respond to their infants at night because of worries caused by events during pregnancy, while others may have difficulty in allowing infants to cry alone at night because of their attitude to the needs of their children. Thus, we believe that for night waking to continue beyond the third or fourth month a constellation of predisposing factors would need to be present. The model consists of the factors outlined in Fig. 8.1; these *predispose* parents to experience their infant's pattern of sleeping and waking as a problem, and to *predispose* an infant to cry when it is awake. In discussing the research on this topic we will consider the way demographic, constitutional and caregiving factors have been found to be related to night waking.

Social factors

Socio–economic status, birth order and gender are variables which are often found to be related to important differences between children. However, in

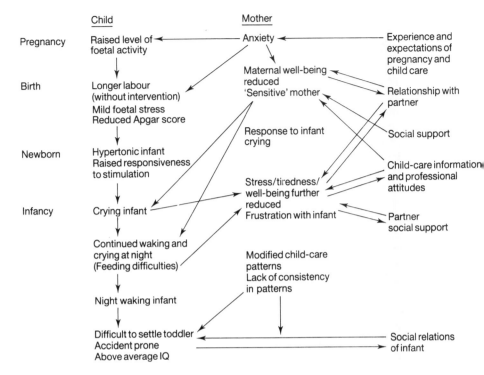

Figure 8.1 Influences on the development of sleep patterns.

the case of sleeping difficulties most studies have failed to detect such relations.

Socio-economic status and ethnic origin

Different types of investigation have consistently failed to find an association between sleeping difficulties or night waking with socio-economic status. For example, Moore and Ucko (1957) in their longitudinal study found no association between the age at sleeping through from midnight to 5 am with father's occupational class, or mother's age or education. The national cohort sample failed to find such differences but admittedly these data were based on retrospective maternal reports about sleeping obtained at five years (Butler and Golding, 1986). Bernal (1973) reports no such difference at fourteen months, although middle-class families were less likely to use a bottle or dummy as a response to night waking. While Scott and Richards (1989) also failed to find that social class and sleeping difficulty were related, they did find that dissatisfaction with housing and overcrowding were related to sleeping difficulties.

Studies using experimenter-identified sleep problem groups have not reported differences according to SES. Similarly, the slightly more complicated definition of sleep problems used by Zuckerman *et al.* revealed no differences according to age of mother, home ownership, social class or overcrowding. However, in this British study differences were found in terms of ethnic origin, sleeping difficulties being more prevalent with mothers from the West Indies or Africa (46 per cent), than from Asia (17 per cent) and the United Kingdom (16 per cent).

Birth order

The birth order of the child has sometimes been found to be associated with sleeping difficulties. Moore and Ucko (1957) report that more first- and second-born children failed to sleep through at thirteen weeks than later born children. Such differences could be the result of differences in parental checking or anxiety levels. Similarly, Richman (1985) reports that an experimenter-defined sleep problem group was more likely to contain singletons than a control group which had no sleep problems. However, other studies have not found this association to be significant, in terms of: age of sleeping through the night (Grunwaldt *et al.*, 1960); membership of a sleep problem group (at eight months (Zuckerman *et al.*, 1987); at fourteen months (Bernal, 1973)) and night waking (Van Tassel, 1985).

Studies using automated recording devices have failed to find any effects of parity during the first year (Thoman and Whitney, 1989; Anders *et al.*, 1985). Thus, if parents report differences in children's sleeping according to birth order this may be due to differences in their own behaviour and attitudes towards infant disturbances. Another factor here that may play a part is the presence of a sibling. One child may wake another who in turn disturbs a parent. Night waking problems are reported more frequently when siblings sleep in the same room (Scott and Richards, 1989).

Sex

Most studies have failed to find a significant association between sex and sleeping patterns. Moore and Ucko (1957) found no difference between boys and girls in age at the first unbroken sleep from 12.00 to 5 am. Another longitudinal study by Jacklin *et al.* (1980) found no differences between boys and girls from 6 to 33 months in rate or stability of sleeping patterns. The studies of Zuckerman *et al.* (1987) of a sleep problem group at 8 months, and Bernal (1973) of a sleep problem group at 14 months, failed to find any difference related to gender. An exception to this general pattern is a study by Van Tassel (1985), which reports that males were more likely to show sleep disturbance ($r = 0.20$) but, as we have commented earlier, the methodology of this study is suspect. Studies using automated recording devices have not found any effects of sex (Thoman and Whitney, 1989; Anders *et al.*, 1985).

Developmental factors

In contrast to demographic factors, developmental factors, such as genetic contribution, perinatal complications and infant temperament have been found to be related to sleeping difficulties. These findings are reviewed in this section.

Genetic factors

Genetic analysis of sleep disturbance in children is sparse. On the basis of probandwise concordance rates in a representative sample of 13-year-old twins, Stevenson and Graham (1988) estimated the heritability sleep problems on the Rutter Parent Scales to be zero. O'Connor *et al.* (1980) also used mothers' reports of specific behaviour problems in twins. They studied a younger sample of 54 monozygotic and 33 same-sex dizygotic twin pairs. The mean age of the twins was 7.6 years. Using a revised version of the Connors scale, they obtained an intraclass correlation for sleep problems of 0.67 for MZ twin pairs and 0.23 for DZ pairs. This gives a heritability estimate in these younger twins of 0.88 for sleep problems. Other studies have data which indicate that sleep problems such as night waking tend to re-occur in the same families. For example, Scott and Richards (1989) report that mothers whose one year olds were waking more than four nights a week were significantly more likely to have an older child with sleeping problems than mothers whose children were not night wakers. Similar results were obtained in a slightly older sample by Richman (1981).

Perinatal experiences

Perinatal factors have often been found to be associated with sleeping difficulties. The longitudinal study by Moore and Ucko revealed that mild asphyxia at birth was associated with a failure to sleep through the night at three months. Bernal (1973) found in a sample of mothers who had unproblematic home births that longer labour, longer time to cry after birth and lower Apgar ratings at birth occurred more often in the parental–defined sleep problem group compared to the rest of the sample. Similarly, Blurton Jones *et al.* (1978) found that problems in pregnancy, delivery and labour were more prevalent in an experimenter–defined sleep problem group at fifteen months. In addition, Richman (1985) reports that an experimenter–defined sleep problem group were twice as likely to have adverse perinatal events, as compared to a control sample which did not have sleeping difficulties.

The findings of Chavin and Tinson (1980) are an exception to this pattern, but it is unclear which of the differences were significant: the largest difference between a sleeping problem and control group was in terms of the likelihood of having an induced birth. Another study which failed to find an effect of birth events was conducted by Van Tassel (1985), but here the measures were based on maternal recall at least fifteen months after the birth.

Birth weight and prematurity

Most studies have failed to find an association between birth weight or prematurity and sleeping difficulties. One exception to this is a report by Campbell (1958), who has drawn attention to a relation between birth weight and the need for night feeding, lower birth weight infants being the ones who were most likely to need to a night feed in the first four months and to continue to wake.

Other studies have failed to find this association, but may employ samples that exclude infants of low birth weight. No relation between age at sleeping through the night and birth weight was found by Grundwaldt *et al.* (1960) or Moore and Ucko (1957), while Zuckerman *et al.* (1987) found their sleep problem group were no different in terms of the number of low-birth-weight infants.

Anders *et al.* (1985) have compared the sleeping of full-term and premature infants matched for conceptual age. The observations were collected by time-lapse video recordings during the first year of the full-term infant's life (see chapter 7). In general, the similarities between the two groups were found to be greater than the differences.

Infant temperament and behavioural organisation

Bernal (1973) reports from the Cambridge longitudinal study that the night waking group were more resistant to passive movements shortly after birth in a neurological examination and showed mild hypertonicity. These babies also responded more quickly to the removal of a teat in a sucking test on day 5. Furthermore, maternal reports of the duration of time in cot during the first ten days was found to be shorter for the sleep problem group. Carey (1974) reports lower sensory threshold in the sleep problem group at six months using the Thomas and Chess questionnaire. Similarly, Weissbluth (1981), using the Carey Temperament Questionnaire, found that mood, adaptability, rhythmicity and approach/withdrawal were correlated with total duration of sleep, with the difficult infants sleeping less. Van Tassel (1985) reports that the Toddler Temperament Scale item of negative mood and adaptability was related to concurrent parental reports of night waking. Retrospective accounts have also supported this pattern of findings. Blurton Jones *et al.* (1978) report a relation between retrospective recall of baby activity and experimenter-defined sleeping difficulties at fifteen months. Richman (1985) found from retrospective reports that an experimenter-defined sleep problem group was more likely to be described as irritable at 0–12 weeks compared with a control group that had no sleep problems.

Moore and Ucko (1957) found no association between colic and waking in the night, nor between amount of crying and night waking. However, Bernal (1973) reports that an experimenter-defined night waking group cried for longer, more often, but for shorter bouts for the first ten days after birth. She interpreted this as reflecting that the babies were more irritable, but admits it could be a product of maternal responses. When the infants were eight and fourteen weeks old Bernal found no difference in evening crying between the night waking group and the rest of the sample.

Maternal depression

At least five investigations have reported that maternal depression is associated with children's sleeping difficulties. However, it is not clear whether the depression is a cause or a consequence of these difficulties. Richman (1985) found a higher rate of maternal depression in an experimenter-defined sleep problem group of toddlers, high stress in the family, and lack of confiding relationship between the spouses, when compared to a control group who did not have sleep problems. Simonoff and Stores (1987) report a high incidence of maternal concurrent depression in a referral group, and also high incidence of paternal depression/psychosomatic symptoms. In addition, Zuckerman *et al.* (1987) found that maternal depression at eight months was associated with persistent sleeping problems at eight months and three years, and they present analyses which suggest that maternal depression is not a product of infants' sleeping difficulties. Van Tassel (1985) reports that night waking identified by parents was related to maternal depression and family stress at a second interview of their sample. Scott and Richards (1989) found that, at twelve months, sleeping difficulties were associated with maternal depression and negative feelings towards the infant.

Other maternal mood characteristics have been claimed to be associated with children's sleeping difficulties. Gottfarb *et al.* (1961) and Ragins and Schachter (1971) both report maternal anxiety is higher with sleeping difficulties.

Caregiving factors

Four inter-related issues are discussed here: parental responsiveness, the introduction of solids, breast/bottle-feeding, co-sleeping, together with the patterns of care associated with all these practices. Discussion of the findings in this area is difficult because of the inter-relation between the different behaviours.

Parental behaviour

Despite the importance attributed to parental behaviour by behavioural management approaches in maintaining sleeping difficulties, few studies have investigated this dimension. Blurton Jones *et al.* (1978) have reported that mothers of an experimenter-defined sleep group at fifteen months were more likely than the rest of sample to pick the baby up at night and then let the child settle. This group were also more likely to pick the child up if it cried and did this quicker than the rest of the sample in an observation of a play session. Interestingly, Blurton Jones *et al.* do not interpret these findings as support for a position which claims sleeping difficulties are a result of parental behaviour, but rather see it as evidence for infant characteristics caused by perinatal experiences affecting both sleeping patterns and parental behaviour. In addition, Van Tassel (1985) argues that her finding of higher rates of reported night waking by mothers who are employed reflects the fact that such mothers have difficulty in dealing with separations. A subsequent questionnaire failed to find this relationship at an older age.

There are indications that parents who have children with sleeping problems are more socially isolated. In the Cambridge longitudinal study (Bernal, 1972) mothers of night waking infants were less likely to go out with their partner and less likely to take their children to see other children. Unfortunately, this study collected no information about maternal mood, as these findings about social life have been associated with higher rates of depression in other research.

Feeding and sleeping

Feeding method
A number of studies have examined the relation between the method of feeding and children's sleeping diffculties independent of other related behaviours. These studies indicate that across the first year there appears to be an association between sleeping difficulties and feeding method, and that the continuation of breast-feeding may be associated with sleep problems. Carey (1975) has reported that at six months significantly more breast-fed than bottle-fed babies had night waking (waking or crying one or more times between midnight and 5 am, for at least 4/7 nights, for at least four consecutive weeks; 52 per cent against 20 per cent), and the effect was even stronger at twelve months (for those infants who continued to be breast-fed, 67 per cent had night waking). Carey discounts the possibility that these effects are due to nutrition, and found no difference in his sample according to temperament or sensory threshold. Instead, he suggests that breast-fed infants may come to expect more attention when they experience any discomfort or waking. Similarly, Zuckerman *et al.* (1987) report that at eight months a sleep problem group contained more breast-fed infants (32 per cent against 15 per cent). Van Tassel (1985) found that infants who continued to be breast-fed were more likely to have sleeping difficulties. She also found that sleeping difficulties were associated with night feeds and sleeping in the parents' bed. However,

the study conducted by Bernal (1973) found no difference in sleeping at fourteen months according to whether or not infants were breast- or bottle-fed, though in the immediate post partum period evening crying was more marked in the breast-fed babies.

Behaviour during feeding
Moore and Ucko (1957) report that difficulties with feeding at three months are associated with failure to sleep through the night. Bernal (1973) failed to replicate these findings in the Cambridge study. Moore and Ucko also identified babies that were always fed at night, sometimes fed, and never fed. At thirteen weeks only 13 per cent of the no-night feed group woke at night, whereas 40 per cent of the variable group woke at night, but this difference was not significant. The variable night feeding group were found to wake significantly more often over the year though this score is somewhat suspect as it may have been influenced by maternal recall. As the authors point out, interpretation of this relation is difficult: it could be seen as due to inconsistent maternal behaviour, or as mothers trying different solutions to a difficult problem. Again, Bernal failed to replicate Moore and Ucko's finding, and she did not find that night feeding at 8, 14 and 20 weeks was associated with later sleep problems (Bernal, 1973).

Bernal (1973) reports that a (experimenter–defined) sleep problem group at fourteen months was fed more frequently for the first ten days after birth compared to the rest of the sample. But she found no difference in sleeping at fourteen months according to whether they were breast- or bottle-fed, or in maternal attitude to feeding schedules, or in feeding difficulties, but the breast-fed infants showed more marked evening crying in the first ten days of life.

Introduction of solids

Is there a relationship between feeding, use of solid foods and sleeping patterns? It is often claimed that a late feed in the evening or the early introduction of solid foods will assist a baby in sleeping through the night. Reisman in 1958 put forward this view in a letter to *Pediatrics*. However, Grunwaldt *et al.* (1960), Moore and Ucko (1957) and Parmelee *et al.* (1964) found no relationship between the onset of sleeping through the night and the age of introduction of solid foods. Furthermore, Beal (1969) reports no simple relationship between calorie intake, birth weight, and rate of weight increase with night waking. Although the introduction of solids does not appear to be associated with sleeping patterns, it is possible that there is some association with changes in the diurnal intake of milk (Wright *et al.*, 1980; Wright, 1988, chapter 5, this volume).

Although the introduction of solids may not in itself influence sleeping patterns, the content of milk and presumably food may have such an effect.

One example of this is a study of whether the amount of tryptophan is associated with newborn sleeping patterns. The availability of tryptophan influences the synthesis of serotonin in the brain. Both substances have been found to influence sleep behaviour in animals and human adults. Moreover, the amount of tryptophan in human breast milk is known to be subject to wide variations. Yogman and Zeisel (1983) have used a randomised double blind procedure to examine the effects of tryptophan and valine (which competes with tryptophan for transmission across the blood brain barrier) on the sleeping of newborns. Infants being bottle-fed were given for their evening feed either a standard formula, tryptophan with high glucose, or valine with low glucose, the concentrations being within limits recorded for human breast milk. When given tryptophan, in comparison to infant formula, the infants entered quiet sleep 20 minutes earlier and active sleep 14 minutes earlier. When the same comparison was made between valine and the formula, the infants entered quiet sleep 39 minutes later and active sleep 16 minutes later. There was no difference between groups in the total time spent in any of the sleep and waking states within the observation period. However, it is not clear whether tryptophan levels are a significant factor in night waking problems.

Recent suggestions have been made that, for a minority of children, sleeping difficulties could be caused by intolerance to cow's milk. The exclusion of cow's milk from the diet of infants who did not respond to a behavioural management approach to treatment (see chapter 10, this volume) resulted in improved sleeping in a programme conducted by Kahn *et al.* (1989). A double blind cross-over challenge with cow's milk resulted in the reappearance of sleeping difficulties.

More generally, we would suggest that all the studies which attempt to relate feeding practices to sleep patterns should be treated with great caution. Many social and psychological factors are associated with choice of feeding method and there are marked historical changes in feeding practices over very brief time periods. Breast-feeding, giving solids or bottle-feeding are at best broad and very variable categories of behaviour.

Feeding, weaning, and co-sleeping

More recent work has focused on the fact that breast-fed babies may be weaned at a later age, fed more often in the night, and be more likely to be taken into their parents' bed. Elias *et al.* (1986) have claimed that breast-fed infants who are weaned later are more likely to wake at night. They argue that the accepted norms for the development of sleeping were published in the 1950s and 1960s when few babies were breast-fed; this is not quite accurate, at least in the case of Parmelee *et al.* (1964), as 26/46 of their sample were breast-fed. Elias *et al.* state that 'most' studies which have considered breast-feeding have not found that it affects night waking, but again as our review indicates this is not accurate.

The study by Elias *et al.* compared the sleeping of infants whose mothers were 'typical American middle class to other women who are atypical in that they belong to La Leche League' (p. 322). This latter group maintains particular close contact with their infants and delays weaning. Sixteen families were observed in each group, the infants were not first borns, and the samples were matched on age, family size and SES. Information was obtained from mothers by sleep diaries in terms of 15-minute time units. The infants in the two groups showed a different pattern of sleeping (the figures reported are the medians for each group). In the SCG (standard care group) the maximum duration of sleep at 2 months was 6.5 hours and in the LLL (La Leche League) group 5.0 hours. The SCG slept for 8 hours at 4 months, while the LLL group did not show any change until 20 months and their longest bout of sleep was often less than 4 hours. The infants in the standard care group had significantly longer bouts of sleeping than infants in the LLL group at all ages except 2 months. In addition, the total sleep remained at 13–14 hours for the SCG, but for the LLL group it decreased from 15 hours at 2 months to 11 hours at 20 months.

Throughout the study significantly fewer infants in the SCG shared their mother's bed. All mothers were breast-feeding at 6 weeks postpartum. Mothers in the standard care group weaned their babies at a median of 12.8 months (total cessation of breast-feeding and lactation), and all but one of La Leche League continued to breast-feed up to 24 months.

A regression analysis was conducted on sleep bout length at 24 months; the variables used were weaning status, sharing a bed, gender, newborn wakefulness, and these variables accounted for 67 per cent of the variance, with sharing a bed and weaning status being significant predictors. It was found that weaned infants slept significantly longer than nursing infants at all ages at which the comparison was possible (7–24 months); nursing infants slept for bouts of between 4–7 hours whereas weaned infants slept in bouts of 9–10 hours. Furthermore, the total sleep of nursing infants was significantly shorter by at least an hour. Weaning was also found to be closely associated with sharing a bed, and except in one case no weaned infant slept in their mother's bed for more than 1 hour a night.

The issue of whether co-sleeping is related to sleeping difficulties has been examined by Lozoff *et al.* (1984). They argue that the American literature for parents is strongly against sharing a bed with a child, but point out this practice is common in other cultures. Despite this, they found co-sleeping was routine in 35 per cent of white and 70 per cent of black families that were interviewed.

A comparison was made between families in which co-sleeping had not been practised in the preceding month (or in which it had been practised in exceptional circumstances) with families which did practise co-sleeping. White families which practised co-sleeping were significantly less likely to have the child fall asleep in bed, more likely to have adult company at bedtime, and to have lower levels of parental occupational skills and education; only one significant difference was detected in the comparisons with black families, but the number of non-co-sleepers was only nine.

Cross-cultural research by Super and Harkness (1982) found a relation between patterns of care and sleeping. They report that infants of the Kipsigis of Kowet, in Kenya, sleep with their mother and can suckle if they wake. In comparison to American babies in the study by Parmelee *et al.* (1964), the Kowet sleep significantly less during a 24-hour period at 16 weeks (12 hours against 15 hours), and have a significantly shorter maximum sleep (4 hours against 9 hours). The authors attribute these differences to the differences between cultures in child-care practices and, in particular, to expectations about night-time behaviour. They might also be attributable to different patterns of weaning and/or night care, and in sensitivity to infant wakening.

Scott and Richards' (1989) study also suggests a link between night waking and sleeping in the same bed or room as the parents. But as with so much of the evidence in this area it is not clear whether bringing a baby into the parents' room or bed is a response to night waking, whether close proximity simply alerts parents to infant waking or whether sleeping in close proximity in some way predisposes infant waking.

Summary

The practices of breast-feeding, co-sleeping and responsiveness to children's needs appear closely connected to each other, and are often associated with sleeping difficulties. The studies which we have reviewed alert us to these relationships, but they do not provide a way of identifying the causal connection between these practices and sleeping difficulties. This can be seen as part of a larger difficulty in establishing what are the factors causing sleeping difficulties.

Overview

Despite different methodologies and different methods of sampling, the findings concerning children's sleeping are reasonably consistent. The most important methodological issue is that parental reports of night waking seem to be dependent on the child either crying when awake at night or being in close enough proximity that the parent is aware that they are awake from movement or suckling. Thus, findings based on parental report are going to be influenced in part by caregiving practices and attitudes.

The other comment that is worth making is that a number of factors which are usually associated with problems during early childhood are not associated with sleeping difficulties. First, social class does not appear to be related to sleeping problems. This is surprising given the fact that there may be different child-care practices according to social class and that lower class families may more often suffer from overcrowding. What makes the finding even more surprising is that studies of this topic have usually relied on parental reports, which in themselves might be expected to be biased by class. Interestingly, differences are found according to the ethnic origin of the mother, suggesting that cultural practices associated with sleeping may be more important than social class in children's sleeping patterns. The sex of the infant does not seem to influence night waking; this is unexpected as typically males are more likely to suffer from health and behavioural problems in childhood. In the case of parity, earlier borns appear more vulnerable than later borns according to parental reports. However, studies which have not used parental reports have failed to find this relationship. Thus, the effects of parity may be mediated by the sensitivity of parents to night waking. The lack of major demographic influences suggests that what may be important for night waking is individual differences of constitution or differences in the care practices that are adopted across a society.

The majority of studies of pre- and perinatal factors indicate that these are associated with parental reports of sleeping difficulties. However, at least in the Cambridge study (Bernal, 1973) such factors are within the normal limits found in obstetrically uncomplicated deliveries. In addition, infant temperament (as assessed by maternal report) has been found to be associated with sleeping difficulties, in terms of sensory threshold, low adaptability, rhythmicity and approach/withdrawal.

Maternal depression has consistently been found to be associated with sleeping difficulties. Zuckerman *et al.* (1987) present evidence which suggests that maternal depression influences sleeping patterns rather than the lack of maternal sleep leading to depression. One process causing this effect might be variability in the depressed mothers' responsiveness to night waking, which would make the waking behaviour difficult to change.

The relation between caregiving aspects of feeding, co-sleeping, weaning and sleeping difficulties is complex, and it is difficult to tease apart the separate influences of each factor on the others. Mothers who breast-feed their infants, who feed them at night, and who sleep with their infants are more likely to report more frequent night waking; the findings about late weaning and the introduction of solids are conflicting, in that most studies have failed to find a relationship but there are some that have. Making sense of the investigations in this field is made more difficult because of the complexity and range of behaviour that can occur. Weaning and the introduction of solids can occur in various ways but has tended to be dealt with as one undifferentiated behaviour. Similarly, co-sleeping can take various forms but tends to be treated as an undifferentiated behaviour. Furthermore, there is an important methodological issue of whether co-sleeping makes the parent more aware of infant waking and so better placed to report it.

To integrate the preceding material we wish to propose a model of children's sleeping difficulties. The model consists of a number of factors, working interactively, which *predispose* parents to report a night waking problem, *predispose* an infant to cry when it wakes at night, and *predispose* parents to reinforce the crying. These can be shown schematically (see Fig. 8.1).

Given a developmental view, night waking cannot be regarded as being caused by a mother or baby. As yet, we have very little independent evidence to suggest that infant characteristics predispose an infant to night waking. In addition, it is important to recognise that there may indeed be a number of paths which lead on to sleeping difficulties, for example some parents may be predisposed to respond to their infants at night because of worries caused by events during pregnancy, others may by disposition be responsive to children and have difficulty in allowing infants to cry alone at night. Furthermore, some infants may develop a pattern of settling themselves into long sleeping bouts at an early age. Future research needs to disentangle these different possibilities by collecting information about maternal dispositions prior to birth, by examining patterns of caregiving and response to night waking, and by collecting uncontaminated information about child characteristics.

References

Anders, T. (1978), 'Home recorded sleep in two and nine month old infants', *Journal of the American Academy of Child Psychiatry*, 17, pp. 421–32.

Anders, T.F., Emde, A. and Parmelee, A.H. (eds) (1971), *A Manual of Standardized Terminology, Techniques and Criteria for Scoring States of Sleep and Wakefulness in Newborn Infants* (Los Angelas: UCLA, Brain Information Service).

Anders, T.F. and Keener, M.A. (1985), 'Developmental courses of night time sleep–wake patterns in full-term and premature infants during the first year of life. I', *Sleep*, 8, pp. 173–92.

Anders, T.F., Keener, M.A. and Kraemer, H. (1985), 'Sleep–wake state organisation, neonatal assessment and development in premature infants during the first year of life. II', *Sleep*, 8, pp. 193–206.

Anders, T. and Sostek, K. (1976), 'The use of time-lapse video recording of sleep–wake behaviours in human infants', *Psychophysiology*, 13, pp. 155–8.

Beal, V.A., (1969), 'Termination of night feeding in infancy', *Journal of Pediatrics*, 75, p. 690.

Beltramini, A.U. and Hertzig, M.E. (1983), 'Sleep and bedtime behavior in preschool-aged children', *Pediatrics*, 71, pp. 153–8.

Bernal, J. (1972), 'Crying during the first 10 days of life, and maternal responses', *Developmental Medicine and Child Neurology*, 14, pp. 362–72.

Bernal, J. (1973), 'Night waking during the first 14 months', *Developmental Medicine and Child Neurology*, 15, pp. 760–9.

Blurton Jones, N., Rossetti Ferreira, M.C., Farquar Brown, M. and Macdonald, L. (1978),

'The association between perinatal factors and later night waking', *Developmental Medicine and Child Neurology*, 20, pp. 427–34.

Butler, N.R. and Golding, J. (eds) (1986), *From Birth to Five* (Oxford: Pergamon).

Campbell, J. (1958), 'Duration of night feeding in infancy', *Lancet*, 1, p. 877.

Carey, W.B. (1974), 'Night waking and temperament in infancy', *Behavioral Pediatrics*, 84, pp. 756–8.

Carey, W.B. (1975), 'Breast feeding and night waking', *Journal of Pediatrics*, 87, p. 327.

Chavin, W. and Tinson, S. (1980), 'Children with sleep difficulties', *Health Visitor*, 53, pp. 477–80.

Coons, S. and Guilleminault, C. (1982), 'Development of sleep–wake patterns and non-rapid eye movement sleep stages during the first six months of life in normal infants', *Pediatrics*, 69, pp. 793–8.

Daws, D. (1985), 'Sleep problems in babies and young children', *Journal of Child Psychotherapy*, 11, pp. 87–95.

Douglas, J. and Richman, N. (1982), *Sleep Management Manual* (Institute of Child Health), revised 1985.

Elias, M.F., Nicolson, N.A., Bora, C. and Johnston, J. (1986), 'Sleep/wake patterns of breast-fed infants in the first 2 years of life', *Pediatrics*, 77, pp. 322–9.

Gottfarb, L., Lagercrantz, R. and Lagerdahl, A. (1961), 'Sleep disturbances in infancy and early childhood', *Acta Paediatrica*, 50, p. 212.

Grunwaldt, M.D., Bates, T. and Guthrie, D. (1960), 'The onset of sleeping through the night in infancy', *Pediatrics*, 26, pp. 667–8.

Guedeney, A. and Kreisler, L. (1987), 'Sleep disorders in the first 18 months of life: hypothesis on the role of mother–child emotional exchanges', *Infant Mental Health Journal*, 8, pp. 307–18.

Jacklin, C.N., Snow, M.E., Gahart, M. and Maccoby, E.E. (1980), 'Sleep pattern development from 6 through 33 months', *Journal of Pediatric Psychology*, 5, pp. 295–303.

Kahn, A., Mazin, M.J., Rebuffat, E., Sottiaux, M. and Muller, M.F. (1989), 'Milk intolerance in children with persistent sleeplessness', *Pediatrics*, 84, pp. 595–603.

Lozoff, B., Wolf, A.W. and Davis, N.S. (1984), 'Cosleeping in urban families with young children in the United States', *Pediatrics*, 74, pp. 171–82.

Moore, T. and Ucko, L.E. (1957), 'Night waking in early infancy: part 1', *Archives of Disease in Childhood*, 32, pp. 333–43.

O'Conner, M.O., Foch, T. and Plomin, R. (1980), 'A twin study of specific behavioural problems of socialisation as viewed by parents', *Journal of Abnormal Child Psychology*, 8, pp. 189–99.

Parmelee, A.H., Wenner, W.H. and Schulz, H.R. (1964), 'Infant sleep patterns: from birth to 16 weeks of age', *Journal of Pediatrics*, 65, pp. 576–82.

Ragins, N. and Schachter, T. (1971), 'A study of sleep behavior in two-year-olds', *Journal of the American Academy of Child Psychiatry*, 10, p. 464.

Reisman, M.C. (1958), 'Feeding of solid foods to infants', *Pediatrics*, 22, pp. 604–5.

Richards, M.P.M. and Bernal, J.F. (1972), 'An observational study of mother–infant interaction', in N. Blurton Jones (ed.), *Ethological Studies of Child Behaviour* (Cambridge: Cambridge University Press).

Richman, N. (1981), 'A community survey of characteristics of one-to-two year olds with sleep disruptions', *Journal of the American Academy of Child Psychiatry*, 20, pp. 281–91.

Richman, N. (1985), 'A double-blind drug trial of treatment in young children with waking problems', *Journal of Child Psychology and Psychiatry*, 26, pp. 591–8.

Scott, G. and Richards, M.P.M. (1989), 'Night waking in infants: effects of providing advice and support for parents', *Journal of Child Psychology and Psychiatry*, 31, pp. 551–69.

Seymour, F.W., Bayfield, G., Brock, P. and During, M. (1983), 'Management of night-waking in young children', *Australian Journal of Family Therapy*, 4, pp. 217–23.

Simonoff, E.A. and Stores, G. (1987), 'Controlled trial of trimeprazine tartrate for night waking', *Archives of Disease in Childhood*, 62, pp. 253–7.

Stevenson, J. and Graham, P. (1988), 'Behavioral deviance in 13 year old twins: an item analysis', *Journal of the American Academy of Child and Adolescent Psychiatry*, 27, pp. 791–7.

Super, C.M. and Harkness, S. (1982), 'The infant's niche in rural Kenya and metropolitan America', in L.C. Adler (ed.), *Cross-cultural Research at Issue* (New York: Academic), pp. 47–55.

Thoman, E.B. and Glazier, R.C. (1987), 'Computer scoring of motility patterns for states of sleep and wakefulness: human infants', *Sleep*, 10, pp. 122–9.

Thoman, E.B. and Whitney, M.P. (1989), 'Sleep states of infants monitored in the home: individual differences, developmental trends, and origins of diurnal cyclicity', *Infant Behaviour and Development*, 12, pp. 59–75.

Van Tassel, E.B. (1985), 'The relative influence of child and environmental characteristics on sleep disturbances in the first and second years of life', *Developmental and Behavioral Pediatrics*, 6, pp. 81–6.

Weissbluth, M. (1981), 'Brief clinical and laboratory observations. Sleep duration and infant temperament', *Journal of Pediatrics*, 99, pp. 817–19.

Wright, P. (1988), 'Learning experiences in feeding behaviour during infancy', *Journal of Psychosomatic Medicine*, 32, pp. 613–19.

Wright, P., Fawcett, J. and Crow, R.A. (1980), 'The development of differences in the feeding behaviour of bottle and breast-fed human infants', *Behavioural Processes*, 5, pp. 1–20.

Yogman, M. and Zeisel, S.H. (1983), 'Diet and sleep patterns in newborn infants', *New England Journal of Medicine*, 309, pp. 1147–9.

Zuckerman, B., Stevenson, J. and Bailey, V. (1987), 'Sleep problems in early childhood: continuities, predictive factors, and behavioral correlates', *Pediatrics*, 80, pp. 664–71.

Chapter 9

Sleep disturbance in children and its relationship to non-sleep behaviour problems

Jim Stevenson, *University of London*

Introduction

This chapter reviews the extent to which sleep disturbance (SD) is associated with other behaviours, particularly problem behaviours. Associations are most usually conceptualised in terms of current co-occurrence of SD and a problem such as daytime non-compliance. However, the associations need not be concurrent, but rather the SD may precede other later behaviour problems or the SD may emerge after other problems have been shown. These associations need not be mutually exclusive, in that the SD may co-occur with one particular problem and be preceded by and/or followed by other problems. In covering this topic it is useful to extend the age range beyond that used by Messer and Richards in their chapter. There are a number of reasons for this: one is the paucity of data from the under-two year olds, another concerns the possibility that links with other behaviour problems may vary with age of the child and there is the possibility that consequences of early SD may only emerge at later ages.

In the studies of SD there are marked variations in the extent to which SD is considered as a 'problem' or thought to reflect some underlying abnormality. Some studies are premised on the idea that SD simply reflects more or less extreme variations in normal child behaviour. Others only study cases where the parents evaluate the sleep behaviour as being problematic for the child and/or the family. Most often there is a researcher-based rating of the severity of the SD that is undertaken in conjunction with data on the frequency of the behaviour.

In reviewing this topic it is often difficult to distinguish the type of SD that is being considered. The majority of studies have centred on night waking as the primary symptom. The second most common problem investigated is that of difficulty in settling to sleep, including 'curtain calling' at bedtime. More specific sleep behaviours have been the subject of a more limited number of studies; these include bruxism (teeth grinding), nightmares, night terrors, sleep walking/talking and co–sleeping. There have been no studies on early morning waking and its relation to other behaviours. It is clear from many studies that these sleep problems tend to co–occur. It is therefore very difficult to tease apart the behavioural correlates of night waking from, for example, those of co–sleeping or settling difficulties. This is a weakness in the literature because, although often co–occurring, different facets of SD in children may well have distinct aetiologies which might be expected to have different correlates in concurrent or subsequent non–sleep-related behaviour (NSRB). This rather clumsy label is used throughout this chapter to refer to other aspects of behaviour that are, like sleep disturbance, often identified as a problem.

In considering the relationship between the NSRB of the child and sleep disturbance, a number of alternative mechanisms could be acting.

$$1.\ \text{NSRB} \rightarrow \text{SD} \qquad\qquad 2.\ \text{SD} \rightarrow \text{NSRB}$$

$$3.\quad X \begin{array}{l} \nearrow \text{NSRB} \\ \searrow \text{SD} \end{array} \qquad\qquad \begin{array}{l} 4.\ X \rightarrow \text{NSRB} \\ \quad\ \updownarrow \\ \quad\ Y \rightarrow \text{SD} \end{array}$$

Here NSRB and SD simply represent a non–sleep-related behaviour and sleep disturbance, which can have causal influences on each other (as in 1 and 2). They might be associated through sharing a common influence, X (as in 3) or may be linked through separate but correlated causes, X and Y (4). At present there are simply too few studies that have been designed to differentiate between these plausible causal models for any firm conclusions to be reached about their relative importance in determining the associations between sleep and NSRB. However, examples that fit the alternative models will be identified.

This review is organised along the following lines. The link between SD and NSRB will first be considered by looking at SD in groups of children where the NSRBs are part of some other condition, for example Rett's syndrome or visual handicap. This is followed by an examination of the co–occurrence of more specific forms of sleep disorder. The co–occurrence with other behaviours will then be examined. The place of sleep in multivariate analyses of problem behaviour in large samples will be considered next. The NSRBs of children identified as SD from clinic referrals and in community surveys will then be reviewed. Finally, an attempt will be made to integrate these disparate studies to form an overview of the processes linking SD and NSRB.

Association between sleep disturbance and non-sleep-related behaviours in children with various conditions

A search using the CD-ROM version of Medline identified a number of studies where SD occurred as part of the clinical pattern in conditions where other distinctive behaviours were also found. The most substantial of these findings are reported here to establish the indications they may provide as to why sleep and NSRB might co-occur.

In a series of three studies Kaplan *et al.* (1987) investigated sleep problems in preschool-aged children with attention deficit disorder and in control children without the disorder. Findings from the first two studies demonstrated clearly that parents of hyperactive children considered their children to have many more sleep problems than did parents of the control children. Parental daily documentation, which is less likely to be affected by reporting bias, was used in the third study. Although the findings showed an increased frequency of night wakings in these children, there was no difference in total sleep time or sleep onset latency between the two groups. The greater number of sleep wakings, which disrupt parents' sleep, may be responsible for the clinical reports that these children are poor sleepers.

In this condition it is possible that the NSRB problem is leading to the SD, i.e. the hyperactive child once awake is more likely to get up or to alert the parents to his or her wakenings. However, Mefford and Potter (1989) have proposed an explanation for the link between SD and attention deficit disorder in terms of physiological differences in adrenaline activity. The consequences are inability to maintain focused attention, difficulty in falling asleep and light levels of sleep.

Kaplan *et al.* (1989) conducted a ten-week study in which all food was provided for the families of 24 hyperactive preschool-aged boys whose parents reported the existence of sleep problems or physical signs and symptoms. A within-subject cross-over design was used, and the study was divided into three periods: a baseline period of three weeks, a placebo–control period of three weeks, and an experimental diet period of four weeks. According to the parental reports, more than half of the subjects exhibited a reliable improvement in behaviour and negligible placebo effects. Alongside these improvements in activity level night waking and settling became less problematic.

One estimate suggests that 20 per cent of visually handicapped children have difficulties falling asleep compared to 6 per cent of a control group (Jan *et al.*, 1977). The most obvious explanation is that the absence of light sensitivity makes it difficult to establish and maintain daily cycles of wakefulness and sleep. This cannot be the whole explanation, since a strong situational effect on these SDs was found by Kitzinger and Hunt (1985). In a sample of 23 visually handicapped 2–5 year olds, the rates of night settling and night waking problems were higher based on the parents' report of sleep behaviour at home (40 and 20 per cent, respectively) than that obtained from reports of sleep at their residential nursery (10 and 5 per cent, respectively). Within this visually handicapped sample there was a high incidence of behaviour disturbance, but there was no significant association between the presence of SD and the other items on the Behavioural Screening Questionnaire (BSQ) (Richman *et al.*, 1982).

Little is known about sleeping in mentally handicapped children. Clements *et al.* (1986) have shown that sleeping difficulties occur frequently in mentally handicapped children of all ages, i.e. in 30 per cent of children under 15 years. There are a number of behaviours that were found to be linked with sleep disorders. These included self–injury, non–socially directed difficult behaviour and attachment to routines. Other behaviours, for example, socially directed aggression, did not show an association. It is difficult to equate these findings with those from non–handicapped children but clearly in both populations SD is not occurring in isolation in a significant number of children.

In other conditions there are anatomical features or illnesses that represent a common cause of SD and NSRBs. For example, sleep apnoea in children develops when airway obstruction at night is severe (Potsic, 1989). The most common cause of night–time obstruction with or without apnoea is hyperplasia of the tonsils and adenoids. Other conditions, such as craniofacial anomalies and neuromuscular disorders, may predispose children to obstruction of the airway during sleep. Apnoea has also been postulated to play a role in some of the behaviour problems seen in Down's syndrome children (Silverman, 1988). However, for the majority of children there is no evidence that apnoea is related to any behavioural problems.

There are a number of medical conditions where SD is found along with NSRB. For example, Rett's syndrome is a progressive disorder that occurs in females and is characterised by autistic behaviour, dementia, ataxia, loss of purposeful use of the hands, seizures and sleep abnormalities. Polygraphic studies have shown abnormal respiratory patterns during wakefulness, and abnormal sleep and electroencephalographic characteristics (Glaze *et al.*, 1987). In Rett's syndrome the co–occurrence of SD and the autistic–like behaviour can be accounted for by the common effects of central nervous dysfunction.

Lacey (1986) has suggested that the combination of chronic motor and vocal tics, Tourette's syndrome, may in some children be associated with thought and behavioural disorders, SD, headaches, and school difficulties (e.g., attention deficit disorder). Comings and Comings (1987) found that sleep problems were pervasive in patients with Tourette's syndrome, with a significantly increased frequency of sleepwalking, night terrors, trouble getting to sleep, early awakening and inability to take afternoon naps as a young child. Jankovic and Rohaidy (1987) and Champion *et al.* (1988) have also demonstrated the high levels of SD in Tourette's syndrome patients where it is found associated with a wide range of disturbed behaviour. In a review of recent research on Tourette's syndrome, Robertson (1989) notes that a number of SDs are consistently reported to be associated with Tourette's syndrome. There is no general agreement as to whether these represent a disorder of arousal in these subjects, but it is most likely that both SD and NSRB are products of disordered brain functioning.

Griffith and Slovik (1989) have drawn attention to the need to consider Munchausen syndrome by proxy as a possible cause of SD. This is a factitious disorder of childhood in which a parent fabricates medical history or produces signs of illness in a child to keep the child in a sick role. Often the parents are found to give the child medication which has an impact on the central nervous system. Approximately half of all cases of Munchausen syndrome by proxy are presentations of central nervous system illness, and include SDs such as excessive daytime sleepiness. These children may show a wide variety of other behavioural symptoms possibly due to other aspects of discordant relationships within the family (Meadow, 1989).

As in adulthood, sleep disturbance is a feature of major depressive disorders. For reviews of aspects of SD in children with depression see Puig-Antich (1987) and McConville and Bruce (1985).

Summary of sleep and non-sleep-related behaviours in children with various conditions

The studies reviewed in this section have provided examples of each of the four models of the association between sleep and NSRB. Model 1, where SD was seen to be in part a consequence of the NSRB, was exemplified by hyperactivity, visual handicap and depression. Model 2 was less frequently found to be operating. Here SD was contributing to the other behaviour problem. One possible instance of this was in Down's syndrome children where the sleep loss and disturbance consequent upon apnoea were thought to contribute to difficulties in daytime behaviour. Rett's and Tourette's syndromes were both examples that fitted model 3 of a common cause (i.e. brain dysfunction). Model 4 is less readily exemplified. However, Munchausen syndrome by proxy is possibly an instance, where sleep and NSRB were caused by independent but correlated aspects of family dysfunction.

The association between SD and certain aspects of psychopathology in children has been reviewed by Garreau *et al.* (1989). They concentrated upon links between more severe forms of psychopathology, such as autism, and organic conditions, such as epilepsy and SD. They attempt to classify the 'dominant pathophysiological mechanisms' producing the specific types of SD. The conclusions they reach concerning the relative significance of 'circadian rhythms,' 'sleep structure' and 'maturation' are not clearly supported by the studies in their review. For the present it is best to treat as conjecture their conclusions, such as that SDs associated with 'psychoaffective disorders' are linked with circadian rhythm alterations, whereas attentional deficit disorder is linked to problems in sleep structure.

Studies of specific sleep-related behaviours

The association of SD and NSRB in children with a range of diagnoses has illustrated the complex patterns of inter-relationships that can be identified. Such an investigation can be taken a little further by looking at the behaviour of children who show specific forms of SD.

Night terrors are a sleep disorder resulting from a partial arousal during slow-wave sleep. They usually occur within two hours of sleep onset and are characterised by agitation and unresponsiveness to external stimuli. DiMario and Emery (1987) studied nineteen children (ten males, nine females) with onset of night terrors before age 7.5 years. Fifty per cent stopped by age 8 years; 36 per cent continued into adolescence. No common abnormal behavioural profile or psychopathology was found. Common precipitants of attacks were not identified.

Rugh and Harlan (1988) have discussed nocturnal bruxism (grinding of teeth) and its relation to disorders of the masticatory system and headaches. Bruxism is believed to be a stress-related sleep disorder, occurring in children and in adults. There is no good evidence for this assertion for children. If stress was significant then it would be expected that bruxism would tend to occur alongside other non-sleep behaviours. There have been no reports of such findings.

In the two cases examined (night terrors and bruxism) there is no evidence of disturbance in other aspects of the child's behaviour.

Multivariate analyses

The previous section concerned less common and rather specific aspects of sleep-related behaviour. It is now appropriate to turn to studies looking at more common forms of SD. This will be undertaken initially by reviewing those studies that have analysed sleep as just one of a large number of potential areas of problem behaviour in children. These studies can be based either on representative samples or on children thought to show a high level of behavioural disturbance. The interest for the present review is to establish whether sleep symptoms are found to be consistently linked with particular patterns or clusters of other behaviours. The analysis of these data can be broadly divided into studies using factor analysis based upon the correlations between pairs of behaviours and those using cluster analysis. In factor analysis the interest lies in seeing if distinct patterns of symptom co-occurrence produce high loadings on common factors. Cluster analysis can be used to identify individuals with similar profiles. Both types of analysis allow us to examine the place of sleep behaviours within naturally occurring symptom clusters.

Factor analysis

Empirically derived classifications of patterns of childhood behaviour have usually included SD. In their landmark review Achenbach and Edelbrock (1978) suggest that sleep problems constitute a separate narrow-band syndrome in their own right and cite as support the studies by Arnold and Smeltzer (1974), Dreger et al. (1964) and Miller (1967). Subsequent studies have identified a rather more complex relationship between sleep and other symptoms. For example, the Child Behavior Checklist (CBCL; Achenbach et al., 1987) has been used by Verhulst et al. (1988) to collect data from 6–11 and 12–16-year-old girls. In the younger girls both 'sleeps little' and 'can't sleep' had a factor loading greater than 0.3 on a schizoid–obsessive factor in samples from both Holland and the United States. In the older age group these items only loaded on an anxious–obsessive factor for the American girls alone.

The factor analysis was based on CBCL scores obtained for girls referred to mental services in the two countries. It is possible that SD in a less deviant population may show a very different pattern of associations with other behaviour. These same reservations hold for parallel data on boys, where sleep was not found to load on any factor at either age in either country (Achenbach et al., 1987).

Soli et al. (1981) used an earlier version of the CBCL with clinic referred samples aged 4–15 years. In boys they found that SD (insomnia) loaded on a factor they called 'somatic regulatory deficit' along with poor motor coordination, speech problems and overtiredness. A somewhat different picture emerged with girls, where insomnia loaded on the 'hyperactivity' factor.

Rutter has grouped sleep difficulties with neurotic items on the basis of the original validation data of the Rutter Parent Scale (Rutter et al., 1970). In that study, SD in middle childhood was found to be associated with neurotic disturbance, especially in girls.

One of the most thorough factor analytic studies on sleep disturbance itself was conducted by Fisher and McGuire (1990). They factor analysed the behaviour scores of 838 unselected 6–12 year olds. They derived a five factor solution within which only one factor ('Bedtime resistance') could be unambiguously labelled.

Cluster analysis

Richman *et al.* (1982) undertook a cluster analysis of the behavioural items from the BSQ with a pooled sample of 183 behaviour problem and control children who were aged three years. Sleep problems did not emerge as a distinctive feature of any of these clusters. However, difficulty in settling at night and waking at night were clearly associated with overall behaviour problems in this community sample.

The Missouri Children's Behavior Checklist was used by Curry and Thompson (1985) in a cluster analysis of psychiatrically referred children aged between 3 and 12 years. Here sleep problems feature only as part of an 'unclassified' cluster.

One of the few other published cluster analyses on preschool behaviour problems is that undertaken by Wolkind and Everitt (1974). They used data based upon the BSQ given to the mothers of three-year-old children and employed the same definition of SD as that of Richman *et al.* (1982). The sample comprised 100 randomly selected nursery school children and a smaller group of 31 children thought to be more at risk of behaviour disturbance. Sleep disturbance was a particular feature in two of the five clusters. The first was a cluster with a high number of behaviour problems centring around sleeping (going into parents' bed and problems going to bed) and eating. They gave the tentative suggestion that this developmental phase related to poor parent–child interaction. The other cluster to include sleep as a feature was a group of essentially normal well-adjusted children. In this group night waking was one of a number of relatively common problems that obtained a high mean score compared to other behaviours within the cluster, but in absolute terms night waking was not a particularly marked feature of the cluster. These two clusters, where sleep-related problems featured, were found to make up 26 and 50 per cent, respectively, of the representative sample of three year olds.

In an analysis of the relationship between temper tantrums and other items of difficult behaviour from the BSQ, Needlman *et al.* (1991) found some specific links with SD. The data were based upon two sources: a general population sample (see Zuckerman *et al.*, 1987) and a sample of children identified by their health visitors as showing some behaviour problems (see Stevenson *et al.*, 1988). The sample consisted of 508 three-year-old children. Multidimensional scaling analysis of the co-occurrence of behaviour problems showed temper tantrums and SD to be closely associated when frequent temper tantrums are present. These two items tend *not* to co-occur when less marked temper tantrums are present. The findings have been summarised in Figures 9.1 and 9.2. In these figures the distance between behaviours is an

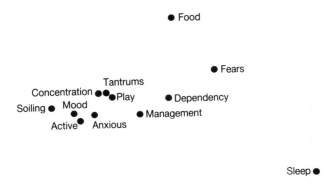

Figure 9.1 ALSCAL analysis two–dimensional solution based upon co–occurrence of behaviour problems in a group where frequent temper tantrums are absent (*n* = 444).

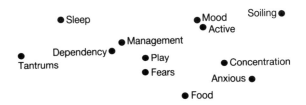

Figure 9.2 ALSCAL analysis two–dimensional solution based upon co–occurrence of behaviour problems in a group where frequent temper tantrums are present (*n* = 56).

index of the extent to which they tend to co–occur. A cluster analysis of these same data also supports this conclusion.

Summary of multivariate analyses of sleep and other behaviours

There is a complex relationship between the occurrence of SD and NSRB. Furthermore, the relationship seems to vary with age and the sex of the children being studied. The idea that SD simply constitutes a separate specific problem (Achenbach and Edelbrock, 1978) has not been supported. There are some preschool children in whom sleep appears as a relatively isolated area of behaviour disturbance. However, sleep problems can also form part of a more extensive behavioural disturbance, which may include temper tantrums.

These complexities make it unsurprising that no clear and consistent pattern of results has been obtained from different factor analyses. The association between SD and NSRB is unstable and will depend on age, sex and severity of overall disturbance. Minor differences between samples in the number of subjects falling into these categories will affect the pattern of association and therefore the derived factor structures.

Studies of the behaviour of sleep-disturbed children

So far, sleep behaviour has been considered as part of the behavioural profile of children with other conditions and the pattern of association between aspects of SD and other behaviours identified by multivariate analyses of data from large samples of normal children. It is time to turn to studies of the behaviour of children that have been identified as having SD.

In considering these data it is sensible to differentiate between studies based upon community samples and those obtained from children referred to clinics. It is well recognised that mechanisms underlying the referral process may distort the conclusions about the characteristics of a particular condition. The significance of such a bias in studies of sleep has been discussed by Messer and Richards (chapter 8). It is also important to consider whether behaviour associated with SD in these studies constitute behavioural precursors, current correlates or behavioural consequences of SD. It is also possible that the pattern of association will be consistent with more than one of these alternatives.

Clinic referrals

Some children who are referred for clinical examination using techniques such as EEG have been reported as showing a variety of NSRB. For example, DeLong *et al.* (1987) report that children referred for sleep EEG and who exhibit the 14 and 6 Hz positive spike phenomenon show high levels of behaviour disorders and aggression. These behaviours include disturbances of temper, mood, attention and learning.

When considering the behaviour problems associated with SD there is some evidence that these associations may be stronger in the general population than in the group referred for treatment. This is illustrated by the treatment sample used by Richman *et al.* (1985). They found the rate of behaviour problems to be 21 per cent in this referred sample compared to the community group of night waking children obtained by Richman (1981), where the rate of behaviour problems was 55 per cent. There is no report of which types of problem behaviour were found in this clinic sample.

Community samples

One of the most systematic attempts to identify the behavioural characteristics of night waking children was the community survey undertaken by Richman (1981). Data were obtained on the sleep and other behaviours of a sample of 771 one to two year olds. Although there was an overall high rate of children with multiple problems in the SD group, they only differed significantly from controls in the percentage of subjects showing food fads (47 against 17 per cent). There was a similar difference in the percentage of night waking children and controls described by their parents as 'irritable' during the first three months postpartum. Interestingly, in this age group temper tantrums were not associated with sleep disturbance. In part this may be due to their relative infrequency during the second year of life.

The Waltham Forest epidemiological study (Richman *et al.*, 1975) provided an estimate of the prevalence rate of sleep and other behaviour problems in a population of urban three year olds. They used the BSQ to assess behaviour problems on the basis of maternal report. There was no particular concurrent association between SD and other specific behaviours. Furthermore, there was no evidence of a link between SD and later problems. For example, in both boys and girls night waking as part of an overall pattern of behaviour problems at three years did not significantly increase the risk of neurotic disorders at eight years (Richman *et al.*, 1982).

Lozoff *et al.* (1985) studied the characteristics of children attending a health clinic for routine appointments, who showed sleep problems. Although an extensive assessment of the childrens' behaviour was not undertaken, they suggest that sleep problems are a significant early childhood symptom of later problems. SDs lasting more than one month are likely to persist and to be associated with maternal ambivalence towards the child, a hospitalisation or accident in the family, maternal depression, mother's return to work and with continuing co-sleeping. These factors, as well as within-child influences, were suggested as possibly leading to a broader disturbance in children. Such an elevated risk of later psychopathology had been claimed in an earlier study by Ragins and Schachter (1971).

A recent epidemiological study in Montreal of 918 three year olds (Larson *et al.*, 1988) has found a similar overall prevalence of behaviour problems (11 per dent) to that identified in the Waltham Forest study (14 per cent) (Richman *et al.*, 1982). This is particularly striking given the nationality differences and the use of a different method of assessing preschool behaviour disorders. Applying the CBCL criteria, the rate of sleep problems in this sample was 3.2 per cent. Of these children 50 per cent showed a high overall behaviour problem score. This percentage of abnormal cases was the lowest of any of the six syndrome groups, and indicates that at three years of age SD is often an isolated behaviour not co-occurring with a wider range of behavioural difficulties. The pattern is also consistent with SD showing significant association with the 'general determinants' of behaviour problems. Larson *et al.* (1988) differentiate general and specific determinants. In each case the determinants linked to SD were very general ones reflecting aspects of stress in the families. Interestingly, at this age SD was not associated with having been breast-fed, paralleling the findings of Zuckerman *et al.* (1987).

Summary of the behaviour of sleep-disturbed children

There is a consistent finding that SD is associated with behavioural problems. This associated is stronger in general population samples than in those children referred for SD. However, the majority of children with SD *do not* show more extensive behaviour problems. When SD is found associated with NSRBs there is no strong evidence from these studies for a specific type of behavioural disturbance to co–occur. Food fads and irritability in the newborn period have been reported as being associated with SD.

Changes in sleep disturbance and in other behaviours

It is now appropriate to turn to findings concerning changes in sleep and other behaviours. It would be of great interest to know whether sleep problems wane alongside changes in other aspects of behaviour and, if so, the relative timing of the onset of such changes. However, none of the published studies provide sufficiently detailed data on the timing of changes in sleep and other behaviours to make any conclusions possible about the relative strengths of the complex causal links between these problems. Nevertheless, longitudinal data do provide one of the most potent insights into the nature of the links between SD and NSRB in children.

Longitudinal studies on sleep disturbance

Garrison and Earls (1985) reported on the continuities in behaviour in a sample of 61 children studied at three and again at six years of age. The findings showed only modest correlations between sleep problems measured on the BSQ at three years and the sleep items on the CBCL at six years. More striking was the association between sleeping problems at three years and broader indices of disturbance at six years (assessed from the Child Behaviour Profile). Sleep problems at three years were significantly correlated ($r = 0.38$–0.47) with schizoid, uncommunicative and somatic complaints factors in boys and with hyperactive behaviour in girls. This is a reversal of the sex difference found by Verhulst *et al.* (1988), where sleep problems were linked to schizoid behaviour in girls but not boys. The correlations of sleep problems at three years with 'internalising' problems at six years was 0.43 for boys and 0.38 for girls. A multiple regression analysis showed sleeping problems at three years to make the single largest contribution to the prediction of both 'internalising' and 'total behaviour problems' at six years.

The follow-up phase of the Waltham Forest study (Richman *et al.*, 1982) allowed an examination in the continuity of sleep problems from the preschool years into middle childhood. Considering the data prospectively, the majority of children with either night settling difficulties, night waking or sleeping in parents' bed at three were *not* doing so at age 8 years. The highest continuity was shown by children in the behaviour problem group, where 48 per cent of those with night settling problems at three also showed such a problem at eight years. A similar picture emerges when the early characteristics of children with sleep difficulties at eight years were examined. Approximately 50 per cent of the SDs at eight years can be seen as continuing from the preschool period. In general, these continuities in SD were greater when they occurred with other behaviour problems at three years of age.

Similar findings were reported by Choquet and Ledoux (1985) in a study of 415 Parisian preschool children. They found that children with many behaviour problems at three years were more likely than matched controls to show SD at seven years of age.

Clarkson *et al.* (1986) studied complaints of sleeping difficulties in a large group of New Zealand children prospectively over four years from five to nine years of age. No association was found between sleeping difficulties and the sex, intelligence or educational attainments of the child. Mothers who described their child as anxious or who were poor sleepers themselves tended to report sleeping problems in their child more frequently. There was no association between sleeping problems and teacher ratings of behaviour problems.

One of the most sophisticated analyses of the characteristics of sleep-disturbed children was that undertaken by Van Tassel (1985). This was a longitudinal study of 70 infants during the first two years of life. There was no significant correlation between SDs reported towards the end of the first year and the end of the second year of life. The only NSRB associated with first year sleep problems was mood. It was suggested that this was in part an artefact of the way the Revised Infant Temperament Questionnaire (Carey and McDevitt, 1978) was scored, where some mood items were concerned with sleep. During the second year both negative mood and low adaptability were related to SD. These two temperamental characteristics were significantly correlated with each other ($r = 0.45$) and mood was related to a number of indicators of family stress and to maternal depression. The variables were entered into two stepwise multiple regressions with sleeping disturbance at each age as the dependent variable. None of the variables related to pregnancy, labour or delivery were significant predictors of SD. The child temperament variables of mood and adaptability were entered in the first step of the multiple regression and between them explain 18 per cent of the variance in year 2 SD. Maternal depression was entered last and explained an additional 1 per cent of the variance after temperament, night-time feeding and parental sleep problems had been taken into account. Breast-feeding was related to SD.

A major difficulty in the interpretation of the results of this analysis stems from the inclusion of aspects of parental management of sleep as predictor variables. Given that these strategies for dealing with SD will have been strongly influenced by the child's sleep history, they would be better considered as consequences rather than causes of SD. Nevertheless, this analysis lends support to the notion that during the first year sleep problems are less a reflection of family stress than those occurring during the second year. This in part accounts for the lack of association between SD at these two time points.

The findings of Van Tassel (1985) were not replicated by Zuckerman *et al.* (1987) in their longitudinal study of 308 children taken from the general population, 56 of which showed SD at end of their first year. When followed up to three years of age, 41 per cent of these 56 children had a sleep problem as measured on the BSQ.

At eight months of age there was only one aspect of NSRB that was associated with SD. Teething problems were more likely in this group (27 per cent) compared to children without SD (14 per cent). Other problems with appetite, bowels or feeding were not related to sleep at eight months. None of these problems, including teething, was related to stability of SD between eight months and three years. Indeed, only maternal depression at eight months was significantly related to sleep disturbance at both ages.

There were a number of behaviours at three years that were significantly more common in the group with persistent SD compared to those with SD at eight months alone. The persistent group were significantly more likely to show poor attention (9 against 3 per cent), to be hard to manage (22 against 0 per cent) and to show frequent temper tantrums (22 against 0 per cent). In this study family factors such as mother's mental state were related *both* to the presence of SD during the first year *and* to their continuity through to three years of age.

The studies by Jenkins and her colleagues at the Thomas Coram Research Unit represent the most extensive continuity data for sleep problems across the whole of the infancy and preschool periods (Jenkins *et al.*, 1980, 1984). They show how frequent night waking peaks during the first half of the child's second year. In addition, the time to time continuity in sleep appears to decrease after the child's second birthday. However, this apparent decline in stability may be an artefact produced by the greater gaps between assessments as the children became older. No details are provided of the co-occurrence of sleep and other problems at any of the ages.

Summary of changes in sleep disturbance and in other behaviours

Longitudinal studies have demonstrated that SDs show modest continuity from infancy into the preschool period. There were similar degrees of continuity between sleep problems at three and eight years of age (though of course these might not be the same children whose SD had persisted from infancy). There are additional associations between SD in the preschool period and a wider range of behaviour problems in middle childhood. The link is not highly specific, although sleep problems at three years were a significant predictor of internalising problems at six years of age as well as one of the best predictors of overall behaviour disturbance at this later age. Finally, there were indications that the continuity in SD between the preschool and middle childhood periods was greater when more extensive behaviour problems were present at the earlier age.

Conclusions

It is clear that SD forms part of the associated behavioural profile of a number of medical conditions. However, there is a distinctive pattern of co-occurrence of SD and NSRB in few of these conditions.

To examine more specific links between sleep and other behaviour, four alternative models were introduced and evidence compatible with all four has been identified. Model 1 – SD may in part be caused by NSRB – was exemplified by hyperactivity, visual handicap and depression. Model 2 – SD contributes to NSRB – was thought to apply to behaviour difficulties in Down's syndrome children. Model 3 – SD and NSRB are both produced by a common cause – was consistent with findings on Tourette's syndrome and this model may also apply to hyperactivity. Model 4 – sleep problems and other behaviours are a product of different but correlated causes – was more difficult to identify. However, it is possible that such a mechanism holds for some children in linking SD and temper tantrums. Needlman *et al.* (1991) have suggested that the temper tantrums are independently associated with a number of family and social factors, such as marital stress, maternal depression and poor child health.

The findings from the studies applying multivariate analyses to behaviours in children in the general population are conflicting. There are differences between age groups and the sexes in the factors which are identified. The results are, however, consistent with the notion that SD can appear as part of a broad profile of behavioural disturbance but also quite commonly as an isolated problem in children who in all other respects are developing normally. One result that needs clarifying is the link found between SD and marked temper tantrums, since in children with less extreme temper tantrums, sleep problems rarely co-occur.

Studies that have looked at concurrent associations between SD and NSRB have identified a number of correlates. These include temper tantrums, food fads, moodiness and attentional deficits. It should be noted that not all studies have found these same behavioural correlates. Whether children with SD are more prone to develop other problems later is less well established. Largely on the basis of retrospective reports there have been claims for links between early SD and behaviour problems in late adolescence. However, prospectively such continuities have only been demonstrated up to the age of eight years.

There is no clear indication of these children being at risk of behaviour problems in later years.

An extensive part of the literature concerns studies of the behaviour of community samples of children with SD. However, such studies have only demonstrated one clear behaviour precursor of later SD, that is measures of irritability during infancy have been related to later night waking, for example in fussing behaviour (Barr *et al.*, 1989), in teething in older infants (Zuckerman *et al.*, 1987) and aspects of early temperament (Richman, 1981).

It would be helpful to be able to distinguish the behavioural correlates of at least night waking and settling difficulties. However, the studies that have looked at associated behaviour problems have rarely presented separate findings for these problems. In part this is due to the common co–occurrence of these two types of SD. It is not therefore possible to test whether night waking might be more closely tied to aspects of the child's physiological functioning during sleep and night settling more related to aspects of parental management.

It is important to re-emphasise that nearly all the research on sleep behaviour has to rely on parental report, so when frequent night waking is studied it concerns those children who wake at night *and* whose parents get to know that they have woken. Children who lie awake without fussing or whose parents are difficult to rouse during the night will not be included in such studies. A parallel issue concerns the parents' acceptance of variation in sleep behaviour in children. Most standardised instruments such as the BSQ have operational definitions of SD based upon frequency of sleep behaviours over a specified period. However, many studies do not use such clear criteria for detecting SD and often rely on parental judgements of the degree to which sleep is problematic. This information on parental assessment of the disruption caused by SD is essential for decisions on the appropriateness of intervention. However, it is less helpful for research purposes. The possibility must be considered in studies using such data that links between SD and NSRB are a reflection of parental expectation or intolerance of the child's behaviour.

Although interest is now developing in the relationship between sleeping, crying and feeding, it is striking that the impact of sleep disturbance on other aspects of the child's development has been so little studied. As well as presenting a disruption to the parents' sleep, disturbance may also result in a state of sleep deprivation for the child. There has been no systematic attempt to identify the consequences of this for the child's growth, arousal or cognitive development. As well as data there is a need for models of how adverse consequences for the child might be manifest, both to guide research but also to aid the planning of intervention.

It can be seen that sleep disturbance can occur both in isolation and in the context of more extensive problems. There are no behavioural correlates that have been consistently found. It would seem that factors within the child, such as irritability, may lead to the association between sleep disturbance and other behavioural problems, such as hyperactivity. Similarly, aspects of parental management might be implicated as in the association between sleep disturbance and food fads. Links with other behaviour problems, such as temper tantrums, might be mediated by aspects both of temperament and parental handling.

There is insufficient data to differentiate between the possible causes of sleep disturbance when it occurs in isolation and when it appears as part of a more extensive profile of behavioural difficulties. It is surprising that there has not been a stronger emphasis in the research reports on possible associations between SD, feeding problems and daytime crying/fussing. Longitudinal studies are required that are designed to investigate all three behaviours and to establish the extent to which they tend to co-occur, whether the pattern of co-occurrence changes with age and to provide tests for alternative models of their aetiology.

References

Achenbach, T.M. and Edelbrock, C.S. (1978), 'The classification of child psychopathology: a review and analysis of empirical efforts', *Psychological Bulletin*, 85, pp. 1275–301.

Achenbach, T.M., Verhulst, F.C., Baron, G.D. and Althaus, M.(1987) 'A comparison of syndromes derived from the Child Behaviour Checklist for American and Dutch boys aged 6–11 and 12–16', *Journal of Child Psychology and Psychiatry*, 28, pp. 437–55.

Arnold, L.E. and Smeltzer, D.J. (1974), 'Behaviour checklist factor analysis for children and adolescents', *Archives of General Psychiatry*, 30, pp. 799–804.

Barr, R.G., Kramer, M.S., Pless, I.B., Boisjoly, C. and Leduc, D. (1989), 'Feeding and temperament as determinants of early infant crying/fussing behaviour', *Pediatrics*, 84, pp. 514–21.

Carey, W.B. and McDevitt, S.C. (1978), 'Revision of the Infant Temperament Questionnaire', *Pediatrics*, 61, p. 735.

Champion, L.M., Fulton, W.A. and Shady, G.A. (1988), 'Tourette syndrome and social functioning in a Canadian population', *Neuroscience and Biobehavioral Reviews*, 12, pp. 255–7.

Choquet, M. and Ledoux, S. (1985), 'La valeur pronostique des indicateurs de risque précoces. Etude longitudinale des enfants à risque à 3 ans', *Archives Française Pédiatrie*, 42, pp. 541–6.

Clarkson, S., Williams, S. and Silva, P.A. (1986), 'Sleep in middle childhood – a longitudinal study of sleep problems in a large sample of Dunedin children aged 5–9 years', *Australian Paediatric Journal*, 22, pp. 31–5.

Clements, J., Wing, L. and Dunn, G. (1986), 'Sleep problems in handicapped children: a preliminary study', *Journal of Child Psychology and Psychiatry*, 27, pp. 399–407.

Comings, D.E. and Comings, B.G. (1987), 'A controlled study of Tourette syndrome. VI. Early development, sleep problems, allergies, and handedness', *American Journal of Human Genetics*, 41, pp. 822–38.

Curry, J.F. and Thompson, R.J. (1985), 'Patterns of behavioral disturbance in developmentally delayed and psychiatrically referred children: a cluster analytic approach',

Journal of Pediatric Psychology, 10, pp. 151–67.

DeLong, G.R., Rosenberger, P.B., Hildreth, S. and Silver, I. (1987), 'The 14 and 6-associated clinical complex: a rejected hypothesis revisited', *Journal of Child Neurology*, 2, pp. 117–27.

DiMario, F.J. Jr and Emery, E.S. (1987), 'The natural history of night terrors', *Clinical Pediatrics (Philadelphia)*, 26, pp. 505–11.

Dreger, R., Lewis, P.M., Rich, T.A., Miller, K.S., Reid, M.P., Overlade, D.C., Taffel, C. and Flemming, E.L. (1964), 'Behavioral Classification Project', *Journal of Consulting Psychology*, 28, pp. 1–13.

Fisher, B.E. and McGuire, K. (1990), 'Do diagnostic patterns exist in the sleep behaviours of normal children', *Journal of Abnormal Child Psychology*, 18, pp. 179–86.

Garreau, B., Barthelemy, C., Bruneau, N., Martineau, J. and Rothenberger, A. (1989), 'Sleep disturbance in children: from the physiological to the clinical', in A. Rothenberger (ed.), *Brain and Behavior in Child Psychiatry* (New York: Springer-Verlag).

Garrison, W. and Earls, F. (1985), 'Change and continuity in behaviour problems from the preschool period through school entry: an analysis of mothers' reports', in J. Stevenson (ed.), *Recent Research in Developmental Psychopathology* (Oxford: Pergamon), pp. 51–65.

Glaze, D.G., Frost, J.D. Jr, Zoghbi, H.Y. and Percy, A.K. (1987), 'Rett's syndrome: characterization of respiratory patterns and sleep', *Annals of Neurology*, 21, pp. 377–82.

Griffiths, J.L. and Slovik, L.S. (1989), 'Munchausen syndrome by proxy and sleep disorders medicine', *Sleep*, 12, pp. 178–83.

Jan, J.E., Freeman, R.D. and Scott, E.P. (1977), *Visual Impairment in Children and Adolescents* (New York: Grune and Stratton).

Jankovic, J. and Rohaidy, H. (1987), 'Motor, behavioral and pharmacologic findings in Tourette's syndrome', *Canadian Journal of Neurological Sciences*, 14, pp. 541–6.

Jenkins, S., Bax, M.C.O. and Hart, H. (1980), 'Behaviour problems in preschool children', *Journal of Child Psychology and Psychiatry*, 21, pp. 5–17.

Jenkins, S., Owen, C., Bax, M.C.O. and Hart, H. (1984), 'Continuities of common behaviour problems in preschool children', *Journal of Child Psychology and Psychiatry*, 25, pp. 75–89.

Kaplan, B.J., McNicol, J., Conte, R.A. and Moghadam, H.K. (1987), 'Sleep disturbance in preschool-aged hyperactive and nonhyperactive children', *Pediatrics*, 80, pp. 839–44.

Kaplan, B.J., McNicol, J., Conte, R.A. and Moghadam, H.K. (1989), 'Dietary replacement in preschool-aged hyperactive boys', *Pediatrics*, 83, pp. 7–17.

Kitzinger, M. and Hunt, H. (1985), 'The effects of residential setting on sleep and behaviour patterns of young visually handicapped children', in J. Stevenson (ed.), *Recent Research in Developmental Psychopathology* (Oxford: Pergamon), pp. 73–80.

Lacey, D.J. (1986), 'Diagnosis of Tourette syndrome in childhood. The need for heightened awareness', *Clinical Pediatrics (Philadelphia)*, 25, pp. 433–5.

Larson, C.P., Pless, I.B. and Miettinen, O. (1988), 'Preschool behavior disorders: their prevalence in relation to determinants', *Journal of Pediatrics*, 113, pp. 278–85.

Lozoff, B., Wolff, A.W. and Davis, N.S. (1985), 'Sleep problems in pediatric practice', *Pediatrics*, 75, pp. 477–83.

McConville, B.J. and Bruce, R.T. (1985), 'Depressive illnesses in children and adolecents: a review of current concepts', *Canadian Journal of Psychiatry*, 30, pp. 119–29.

Meadow, R., (1989), 'ABC of child abuse: Munchausen syndrome by proxy', *British Medical Journal*, 299, pp. 248–50.

Mefford, I.N. and Potter, W.Z. (1989), 'A neuroanatomical and biochemical basis for attention deficit disorder with hyperactivity in children: a defect in tonic adrenaline mediated inhibition of locus coeruleus stimulation', *Medical Hypotheses*, 29, pp. 33–42.

Miller, L.C. (1967), 'Louisville Behavior Checklist for males aged 6–12 years', *Psychological Reports*, 21, pp. 885–96.

Needlman, R., Stevenson, J. and Zuckerman, B. (1991), 'Psychosocial correlates of severe temper tantrums', *Journal of Developmental and Behavioral Pediatrics*, 12, pp. 77–83.

Potsic, W.P. (1989), 'Sleep apnoea in children', *Otolaryngologic Clinics of North America*, 22, pp. 537–44.

Puig-Antich, J. (1987), 'Sleep and neuroendocrine correlates of affective illness in childhood and adolescence', *Journal of Adolescent Health Care*, 8, pp. 505–29.

Ragins, N. and Schachter, J. (1971), 'A study of sleep behavior in two year old children', *Journal of the American Academy of Child Psychiatry*, 10, pp. 464–80.

Richman, N. (1981), 'A community survey of the characteristics of one to two year olds with sleep disruptions', *Journal of the American Academy of Child Psychiatry*, 20, pp. 281–91.

Richman, N., Douglas, J., Hunt, H., Lansdown, R. and Levere, R. (1985), 'Behavioural methods in the treatment of sleep disorders – a pilot study', *Journal of Child Psychology and Psychiatry*, 26, pp. 581–90.

Richman, N., Stevenson, J. and Graham, P. (1975), 'Prevalence of behaviour problems in three-year-old children: an epidemiological study in a London borough', *Journal of Child Psychology and Psychiatry*, 16, pp. 277–87.

Richman, N., Stevenson, J. and Graham, P. (1982), *Preschool to School: A behavioural study* (London: Academic).

Robertson, M.M. (1989), 'The Gilles de la Tourette syndrome: the current status', *British Journal of Psychiatry*, 154, pp. 147–69.

Rugh, J.D. and Harlan, J. (1988), 'Nocturnal bruxism and temporomandibular disorders', *Advances in Neurology*, 49, pp. 329–41.

Rutter, M., Tizard, J. and Whitemore, K. (1970), *Education, Health and Behaviour* (London: Longmans).

Scott, G. and Richards, M.P.M. (1989), 'Night waking in infants: effects of providing advice and support for parents', *Journal of Child Psychology and Psychiatry*, 31, pp. 551–69.

Silverman, M. (1988), 'Airway obstruction and sleep disruption in Down's syndrome', *British Medical Journal*, 296, pp. 1618–19.

Soli, S.D., Nuechterlein, K.H., Garmezy, N., Devine, V.T. and Schaefer, S.M. (1981), 'A classification system for research in childhood psychopathology: Part 1. An empirical approach using factor and cluster analyses and conjunctive decision rules', in B.A. Maher and W.B. Maher (eds), *Progress in Experimental Personality Research, vol. 10* (New York: Academic), pp. 115–61.

Stevenson, J., Bailey, V. and Simpson, J. (1988), 'Feasible intervention in families with parenting difficulties: a primary preventive perspective on child abuse', in K. Browne, C. Davies and P. Stratton (eds), *Early Prediction and Prevention of Child Abuse* (Chichester: John Wiley), pp. 121–38.

Van Tassel, E.B. (1985), 'The relative influence of child and environmental characteristics on sleep disturbances in the first and second years of life', *Developmental and Behavioral Pediatrics*, 6, pp. 81–6.

Verhulst, F.C., Achenbach, T.M., Althaus, M. and Akkerhuis, G.W. (1988), 'A comparison of syndromes derived from the Child Behaviour Checklist for American and Dutch girls aged 6–11 and 12–16', *Journal of Child Psychology and Psychiatry*, 29, pp. 879–95.

Wolkind, S.N. and Everitt, B. (1974), 'A cluster analysis of the behavioural items in the preschool child', *Psychological Medicine*, 4, 422–7.

Zuckerman, B., Stevenson, J. and Bailey, V. (1987), 'Sleep problems in early childhood: continuities, predictive factors and behavioral correlates', *Pediatrics*, 80, pp. 664–71.

Chapter 10

The treatment of sleeping difficulties

David Messer, *University of Hertfordshire*

As has been shown in the previous chapters, children's sleeping difficulties are an important issue for many parents. Health visitors and doctors comment that such issues are assuming an increasing prominence in their case loads. Similarly, the publication of a number of recent books which provide advice for parents in dealing with children's sleeping problems points to the importance of this topic (Daws, 1985b; Douglas and Richman, 1984; Ferber, 1986) and the needs of parents for advice. Parents have often been advised that their child will grow out of the problem; such advice used to be common and is still given. In addition, treatment has involved the use of drugs. As has already been discussed, sleeping problems appear to persist until at least the school years. Furthermore, as we shall see, the use of drugs does not appear to produce improvements over the long term. The ineffectiveness of both these strategies points to the complexity of the organisation of sleeping; for some children maturation on its own does not seem to remove night disturbances, nor does the aid of drugs set up a pattern which children will keep to once the drug treatment is removed.

More recently, the behavioural management approach to dealing with night disturbances has become widely accepted. This approach has progressed from the extinction method, where parents were asked to leave the child to cry, to more gradual and less confrontational methods. A number of investigations have evaluated the success of these methods. Interestingly, treatment in the psychoanalytic tradition tends to utilise similar techniques, although it has a different theoretical orientation.

This chapter brings together a review of the main methods of treating sleeping difficulties in preschool children, together with a description of studies concerned with the evaluation of the effectiveness of treatment. Four methods are examined: drug, behavioural management, information/support and psychoanalytic.

Drug treatment

Although Ousted and Hendrick (1977) have reported that by 18 months a quarter of all firstborns have been given sedatives to help their sleeping, the effectiveness of such treatment is often doubted. Chavin and Tinson (1980) found that 71 per cent of infants who were judged to have serious sleep problems were given drugs, and 55 per cent of the parents who used drugs reported that they had helped on one or two nights, but only 11 per cent said that drugs had been of any help in the longer term.

A study of the use of drugs by Russo *et al.* (1976) compared the effects of using diphenhydramine with that of a placebo. The drug was given for a week and the study involved 50 2 to 12 year olds. They found that the drug reduced the time taken to fall asleep and the number of wakings but did not affect the total time asleep.

Richman (1985), using a double blind procedure, examined the effect of trimeprazine tartrate. The families who took part in this study were volunteers who were identified from a questionnaire survey rather than referrals as is more typical in treatment studies. The drug was administered for two weeks. All families kept sleep diaries. The drug group parents were significantly more likely than the placebo group to report improved falling asleep, night waking and appetite. The number of nights woken was found to be lower when taking the drug than during the baseline period (3.7 against 5.2/week), but this was not true for the placebo group. However, Richman points out that the extent of improvement was limited. Furthermore, at a six months follow up there was no significant improvement from pre-treatment baseline for the drug group on a composite score. Richman also comments that there was no evidence from her study that the use of the drug was effective in improving the child's sleeping habits.

Simonoff and Stores (1987) in another study using a double blind assessment of trimeprazine tartrate found that the drug reduced night waking and prolonged night-time sleep during treatment. However, like Richman they found no difference between the baseline level of night disturbances and the level when the drug was no longer administered.

These well-controlled investigations suggest that drug treatment on its own is not effective. The ineffectiveness of drug treatment has led Douglas and Richman (1982) to recommend that drugs should be seen as a way of giving relief during crises. Even in such circumstances, they recommend that drugs should be complemented by a behavioural management programme.

Behavioural management approaches

In child care books Illingworth (1987), Spock (1969), Valman (1989) and Leach (1989) have all recommended that infants should be left to cry at night. This technique is assumed to work because children's crying will no longer be reinforced by parental attention, and this will lead to the extinction of the crying response. Leach suggests a modified extinction procedure in which parents are recommended to check their child every five minutes but not to interact with them. More recent behavioural approaches also recommend less drastic approaches.

A comprehensive sleep management manual which describes the use of behavioural techniques has been produced by Douglas and Richman (1982; see also Douglas and Richman, 1984). Douglas and Richman emphasise that all treatment programmes should be adapted to the capacities and requirements of the families rather than applying a single method to all cases. They also point out that many families, although motivated by the debilitating effect of continuous sleep disturbances, will be anxious about procedures which may make the child feel unloved. Douglas and Richman state that such parents should be reassured that it is possible to be firm about a child's behaviour while still providing a stimulating and loving environment. In particular, it is often important to say that a family that is well rested can provide a much better environment for a child than one whose members are tired and irritable. Breast-feeding may also be an issue which needs to be discussed with the mother and if she wishes to end night-time feeds or wean the child, then these goals can be integrated with the other treatment.

Douglas and Richman argue that it is not necessary to know the aetiology of sleep disturbance for effective treatment because the parents' responses are likely to be the most important factor in maintaining the disturbances. In particular, sleep difficulties are seen as largely due to the inability of infants who wake up to settle by themselves. However, attention is drawn to the possibility that sleep problems are a product of general difficulties within the family and can reflect marital estrangement. In such cases there would need to be more general treatment and counselling.

The goals of treatment are set by the parents rather than the therapist; the therapist merely ensures that the objectives are reasonable. The therapist's role is to discuss with the parents methods of obtaining the goals and to make sure that the parents believe that they can carry out the programme. Writing down the goals can be helpful in maintaining the programme. It is recommended that both parents attend treatment sessions; this minimises the possibility that one partner will attempt to sabotage the treatment. If possible, the child should be included in these discussions. Douglas and Richman summarise the treatment process as follows:

1. Behavioural analysis of the sleep problem.
2. Analysis of other family problems and parental emotional state.

3. Discussion about the possibilities of change and the parents' feelings about the difficulties they face.
4. Discussion of the possible mechanisms producing settling and waking problems.
5. Encouragement of both parents to attend sessions.
6. Negotiation and agreement about target setting.
7. Discussion of different techniques for change. Use of drugs.
8. Agreement of programme and contract for attendance and sleep diaries.
9. Carrying out the programme and monitoring progress.

Douglas and Richman identify four techniques for change: extinction, positive reinforcement, shaping and graded approaches, and antecedent conditions and discrimination learning. These are only outlined here; for a more extensive discussion see Douglas and Richman (1982, 1984).

Extinction

This involves removing any reinforcing responses to children's behaviour (i.e. ignoring a child who cries in the night). Although this technique can be very effective and fast it can be very upsetting to some parents and children. Furthermore, parents who are referred for treatment are often unwilling to use such a technique or have used it in the past intermittently with the result of partially reinforcing long periods of crying and thereby making the behaviour more resistant to extinction. A slightly less drastic form of using extinction is for a parent to settle the child very briefly with the minimum of interaction, and then go back to check and carry out the process again if necessary five minutes later. Douglas and Richman report that some parents find this approach helpful and it reduces their worries about leaving their child, while others find that it makes the problems worse. Douglas and Richman state that extinction techniques can be used if the child comes into the parents' bed or comes downstairs; the child is simply put back in their own bed with the minimum of interaction and this is repeated for however many times necessary. In such cases, parents should be warned that the methods can be exhausting initially, because of the need to continuously repeat the technique, and it should be stressed that the whole treatment programme will be seriously undermined if they give in to the child's demands at any point.

Positive reinforcement

With older children who have a verbal age of three years or above it is possible to use positive reinforcement to reward desired behaviours with such things as star charts (obviously the reinforcement that is chosen needs to be rewarding to the particular child). The child's maturity makes it possible to make explicit what is expected and what they will receive if they comply with the expectations. When employing this technique it is recommended that reinforcement should be given for carrying out an activity rather than not carrying out an activity (i.e. for staying in bed rather than for not getting up), that reinforcement should never be taken away once awarded, and that when a goal has been agreed it cannot be changed or the criteria for success moved. A disadvantage of this approach is that it is often difficult to give immediate reinforcement for the desired behaviour. If a child fails to achieve an objective then parents should say why he or she is not being rewarded without being angry and make plans for success on the following evening. Praise and congratulations should accompany the award of reinforcement so that these will come to replace the more physical rewards. Usually, the administration of awards becomes unnecessary. In some cases children continue to request a reward when the target behaviour has been achieved; to end such requests the criteria needed for reward can be raised so that the child loses interest.

Shaping and graded approaches

This involves reaching the desired goal in a number of small steps. Douglas and Richman write that this is the most frequently used approach in treatment because parents who seek advice are often not able or willing to carry out an extinction programme. However, shaping takes longer and is more vulnerable to regression to earlier problems. Because of this, careful monitoring, as well as the provision of support, are needed. The technique should also minimise interaction so as not to provide reinforcement for undesired behaviour. Examples are gradually moving bedtimes, or gradually physically distancing the parent from the child at bedtime so that they will eventually fall asleep by themselves.

Antecedent conditions and discrimination learning

This approach seeks to have children associate sleeping and settling themselves with certain events or conditions. The establishment of bedtime routine are an obvious example of this. Douglas and Richman write that, in some cases, where there is no clear routine, a parent may be the cue for sleep rather than the bed or cot. As a consequence, the child will have difficulty settling if they wake and the parent is absent. In such cases it is recommended that children be put in their cot when they are drowsy and need a daytime nap; in this way they will associate going to sleep with the cot and perhaps some toy or music when employed as additional cues.

The effectiveness of the behavioural-management approach

An investigation by Sanger *et al.* (1981) appears to provide one of the earlier investigations of treatment. The therapists were health visitors who met regularly every fortnight with a child psychiatrist. The families receiving treatment were referred by health visitors. Treatment began with the health visitor collecting details about the family and the problem; the parents then kept a diary of sleeping for two weeks. These data were then discussed by the full group at fortnightly sessions and plan of action was formulated. After this, the health visitor usually went to see the mother to give advice about treatment which took into account the ideas of the parent(s). Treatment was not continued in a systematic manner but parents with continuing difficulties were seen again. Four months after the initial questionnaire was completed, a second one was filled in by the parents.

The behavioural techniques that were employed included: extinction, reinforcement, shaping, cuing and fading (gradually reducing a behaviour). Sixteen children had treatment (aged seven months to five years). Before treatment, many parents appeared confused about how to solve the sleeping problems and these problems were having a detrimental effect on family life. The treatment was reviewed on the basis of the four month questionnaire. Nine out of the sixteen were considered to show 'much improvement,' in five cases there was 'little' or 'no improvement' (but in two of these cases the situation was no longer considered a problem by the parents), and no children were considered to have become worse. The authors consider a crucial feature of this treatment plan was the facility to discuss cases with colleagues, and an essential element was the presence of the child psychiatrist at these discussions.

Jones and Verduyn (1983) provide another example of the assessment of behavioural treatment. Their assumptions about treatment were that it should involve: (1) careful analysis of the problem in terms of the behaviours which reinforce the continuation of sleeping difficulties; (2) establishment of goals of treatment; and (3) use of gradual steps to attainment.

Their study examined nineteen children who were up to five years old, and had one or more of the following characteristics: would not fall asleep in bed by themselves, woke at least three times a night, woke for at least an hour a night, or waking and then sleeping in the parents' bed.

In the first interview a general history of the family's health was obtained as well as a detailed history of the sleeping disturbances. Parents were asked to keep a diary for a week. At the first treatment session the diary was discussed, behavioural causes of the difficulties were outlined and the goals of treatment were identified. The goals set for all children included: (1) settle and sleep in own bed; (2) remain in own bed, and (3) not wake parents except in exceptional circumstances.

The way that each goal could be attained was agreed with the parents and typically involved a series of small steps which would gradually stop adult actions which were reinforcing the child's sleeping pattern. Emphasis was placed on the importance of maintaining consistency when responding and parents were warned that problems could become worse before they became better.

For the whole sample, treatment sessions occurred every week until there was clear progress, and then sessions were given every two weeks. The average number of treatment sessions was 5.5. The authors report that at the end of treatment 53 per cent of the children's sleep problems were resolved, 37 per cent showed partial resolution and 10 per cent were unchanged. Six months later the figures were very similar. It was found that the problems were less likely to be resolved if there was marital discord, and joint attendance by parents at the sessions was associated with significantly more effective treatment.

Richman *et al.* (1985) in their assessment of behavioural treatment comment that the method has some drawbacks. These are as follows: that independent assessment of progress is difficult, parental behaviour needs to be modified at night when they are the least alert, the therapist cannot provide model behaviour for the parents and it is usually difficult to use positive reinforcement.

The children taking part in the study were one to five year olds who had a sleep problem for at least six months and the problem occurred at least four times a week (if there was a settling problem this had to last an hour, if a waking problem this had to occur more than three times per night or for longer than twenty minutes, or the child went regularly into the parents' bed). Treatment consisted of six sessions over six months and all families kept a sleep diary before and during the study. At the first diagnostic interview no advice was given and parents were asked to continue keeping a sleep diary (begun two weeks before the diagnostic interview). At the first treatment session the therapist explained the assumptions of the study and that parents could change their child's sleeping by changing their responses. The therapists and parents then agreed on a set of goals.

The original sample consisted of 64 families. Twenty-nine families did not enter treatment; of these 7 had already improved by the first treatment session, and 15 failed to come for the diagnostic or treatment session. The remaining 35 children who entered treatment were between 12 and 48 months old. Five of the families terminated treatment and in these cases improvement was minimal. Of the remainder, 90 per cent were considered to have shown a marked or complete improvement (in the opinion of two members of the treatment team who examined diaries and parental reports). This was maintained four months later except in one case.

Weir and Dinnick (1988) evaluated the effectiveness of using Douglas and Richman's (1982) *Sleep Management Manual* as a basis for health visitors to run a treatment programme. The health visitors collected information from parents in an initial interview and questionnaire and this information was discussed by the group of professionals to identify a course of treatment for each family. The treatment was carried out by a health visitor. The families were followed up six months after the initial interview with another interview and questionnaire conducted by the health visitor. The health visitor rated the severity of the sleeping problem and a clinical rating was made on the basis of questionnaire answers.

A control group of health visitors met a separate research worker who explained the purpose of the study. Health visitors in this group were to conduct identical initial follow-up sessions with the parents. They were also told that they '*should give advice or refer according to their normal practice*' (p. 358, italics added).

The final sample consisted of 42 families, with children between 4 months and 4.5 years (mean 20 months). Both treatment and control groups showed considerable improvement over the six months and no significant differences were detected between the treatment and the control groups. 59 per cent of the treatment group were considered to have a mild or no problem at the end of treatment; 42 per cent of the control group were considered to fall into this category. More children were referred to other agencies in the control group than the treatment group (41 against 8 per cent), but this difference was not significant.

A number of studies of the treatment of night waking have been conducted by Seymour and his colleagues. An early study in this series involved improved organisation of bedtime routines and the minimising of rewards for calling out or for getting out of bed (Seymour *et al.*, 1983). The study was undertaken between 1979 and 1981 and involved 208 families. The children were under six years of age with the majority being under three years of age. Various measures were obtained from sleep diaries, such as time to bed, time to settle, times awake during the night and time taken to go back to sleep. This information was collected prior to, during and after treatment. The treatment involved six items:

1. Questions were asked about sleep patterns, illnesses, etc.
2. Questions were asked about parental expectations, with unrealistic expectations being discussed. Information about normal sleep requirements was given if necessary and the effects of poor sleeping commented upon.
3. Sleeping difficulties were explained in terms of habit learning. Parents were given the impression that they were not the cause of sleeping difficulties but could be responsible for its maintenance.
4. It was explained that sleep difficulties were associated with a lack of bedtime routine, parents being present when children fell asleep, and parents going to children when they woke at night and staying with the child until he or she went back to sleep.
5. The previous success of the programme was emphasised.
6. A general programme was set out with a bedtime routine: the parent to stay briefly with the child when they were put to bed, to ignore crying, and if necessary to put the child back to bed with the minimum of interaction. It was suggested that the parents should in some circumstances shut the bedroom door until the child was quiet. For older children reinforcements for sleeping through the night were suggested.

The parents were given written instructions after a verbal presentation and daily telephone calls were made to follow up on progress. From the start of the programme progress was checked with a second interview one week later, and phone calls were made at two weeks, three weeks, one month, three months and six months.

Seven per cent of the families did not implement the programme. For the remaining sample, the mean number of nights per week when the child woke was reduced from seven per week in the pre-test condition to approximately four per week after one week of treatment, and to approximately one per week, a month after the start of treatment. A follow-up interview on 48 families revealed that about half reported that the child reverted to sleeping difficulties after the initial improvement, and the parents reported that in 70 per cent of these cases they managed to reverse the decline. In addition, nearly three-quarters of the families reported that they 'noticed positive changes in ... daytime behaviour,' and over three-quarters said they were 'happy with ... child's sleep pattern'.

The authors defend their recommendation that parents ignore children's crying. They point out that 95 per cent of parents did manage to carry this procedure out, and argue that parents are able to do this if adequate assurance and daily telephone support is given to them. In addition, the authors tend to discount any harmful effects of this procedure when judged against the positive benefits to families.

Seymour (1987) has also reported the treatment of four cases. The investigation involved a multiple-baseline design across subjects, and reported reasonable success. A more recent larger scale investigation involving a random assignment to treatment and control groups has been conducted by Seymour *et al.* (1989). This study will be considered in more detail in the section on 'information and support' below. However, it is worth noting here that the treatment programme children slept better than the control group after treatment, but that there still continued to be some night disturbance in the treatment group.

Organisation and timing of sleeping

A variation on the usual management approach has been provided by Largo and Hunziker (1984) who emphasise the need for bedtime to take into account the total amount of sleep an infant has during a 24-hour period. Largo and Hunziker used a treatment schedule involving three sessions. At the first session parents are instructed about keeping a sleep chart to describe their child's behaviour in the next 10–14 days. Details about previous history of sleeping are obtained and a routine clinical examination of the child is conducted. In their procedure it is emphasised that both parents should attend the sessions. In the next two visits counselling is conducted using the following principles:

1. Sleep is a highly organised activity which is under maturational control and as a result the pattern is unlikely to be accelerated by the use of solid food or drugs.
2. It takes at least one to two weeks before treatment has an effect.
3. There is large variation in sleeping patterns between infants.
4. The total duration of sleep in a day is usually constant for a child and is biologically determined.
5. The duration of night-time sleep is negatively correlated with that of daytime sleep.
6. Bedtime and awakening time are positively correlated.
7. Night waking occurs in 40 to 60 per cent of infants and therefore is normal.

Of these the most important assumptions appear to be that the total amount of sleep cannot be changed and that the amount of night-time sleep will be influenced by the time children are put to bed and whether they have slept during the day. Bearing these assumptions in mind the parents (and not the therapist) were asked to:

1. Estimate the child's sleep per day.
2. Decide on whether there is a need for a daytime sleep.
3. Set bedtime, bearing in mind that the time in bed should not be longer than the total sleep needs.
4. Keep this schedule for 10–14 days and keep a sleep chart.

Treatment was kept to three visits over a six-week period. An investigation was conducted into the effectiveness of this method of treatment with 52 children aged between 2 and 36 months who were referred to the Swiss outpatient clinic. Largo and Hunziker report that 38 per cent of the families solved the sleep problems by themselves while using the sleep diary and before detailed counselling. The authors suggest this may be because the sleep diary forced caregivers to become better observers of their children's behaviour, with the consequence that they developed more realistic expectations about the amount of sleep. Counselling was undertaken with the remaining families. Typical issues covered were: dealing with unrealistic expectations about the amount of sleep, i.e. parents would often put children to bed early so that they would inevitably not need to sleep through the night. Another common problem was parents expecting changes on one day to have an immediate impact, and anxieties in caregivers of children at risk or of those with health problems.

The treatment procedure was succesful with 85 per cent of the families. In the unsuccessful cases there were additional difficulties associated with the child and/or parents. Successful treatment had a fairly loose definition in terms of age–appropriate sleeping, and it is not clear whether this was based on general parental report or more detailed diary data.

The provision of information and support

The possibility that information and support might reduce sleeping difficulties has been investigated by Scott and Richards (1989). They used three
treatment conditions: (1) the provision of an advice booklet and three support
visits where there could be a non-directive discussion of night waking. Parents
were aware that these visits were not conducted by a trained counsellor or
therapist; (2) the provision only of an advice booklet; and (3) no extra
provision. A further control group was included of families who did not
consider themselves to have an infant with sleeping difficulties. The advice
booklet gave both general information about sleep and an evaluation of the
advantages and disadvantages of various forms of treatment. The aim was to
encourage parents to choose the treatment best suited to them and to bear in
mind perspectives from other cultures.

The infants were less than 18 months old and were mostly referred by
health workers. Thirty infants were randomly assigned to each of the three
treatment conditions. Seventy additional families were referred but did not
enter the study; 50 of these when contacted said that their baby's sleeping was
no longer a problem. The three groups were studied for three months: an
initial interview was conducted; the parents completed four sleep diaries; and
a final interview was conducted. At the interviews the General Health
Questionnaire and the Irritability and Anxiety Scale were administered.

No differences were found at the beginning or end of the study between the
three conditions in terms of parental reports of night waking. The GHQ scores
were significantly higher for the 'booklet and support group' than the other
groups at the end of the study (i.e. the mothers felt less well), but there was no
significant difference between treatment groups when difference scores were
computed. Nor was any difference found between groups in the parental
reports about whether their child's sleeping had improved (depending on
condition, 71 to 82 per cent said there was improvement). However, it is worth
noting that the actual differences in sleeping reported between the first and last
interviews were not large. In discussing these findings, Scott and Richards
point out that other forms of advice or support may be effective, and that their
interventions might be effective as a form of prevention.

Another study by Seymour *et al.* (1989) randomly allocated 45 families to
three groups: a group following a therapist-based treatment programme with
follow-up telephone calls, a group provided with only a simple written guide
with no follow-up telephone calls, and a waiting list control group. The
effectiveness of treatment was assessed from parental reports before and after
treatment. The parental reports were obtained from sleep diaries and an
interview. The children were aged between 9 months and 5 years (mean 18
months). Both treatment groups were found to significantly improve
according to the number of wakings per week (in the full treatment group
there was a change from 16 to 7 wakings; in the written information group a

change from 12 to 5 wakings; and in the control group a change from 13 to 12 wakings). The authors observe that there were wide individual variations in sleep, and it is worth noting that children were on average still waking once a night. The authors comment that the written guide appeared to be as effective as therapist-based treatment but that the effects were not as immediate.

Psychoanalytic perspectives

Guedeney and Kreisler (1987), in examining the characteristics of families with children who have sleeping difficulties, have commented on the high incidence of anxiety, stress and depression in mothers before and after the birth of the child. They 'propose an association between a very active, excited child, a mother–child relationship characterized by hyperstimulation, a mother with many phobic concerns about the child, and subsequent sleep disorders', and they argue that treatment should involve not just the child and the mother, but sometimes the whole family. Such a perspective stands in contrast to the behavioural management approach which tends to treat the issue of sleeping difficulties as a discrete problem.

Daws (1985a, b) has discussed the method she employs to treat children's sleeping difficulties. She suggests parents may often feel that they cannot manage issues connected with sleeping and that in a number of cases the problems can be solved after one or two sessions. The sessions involve structured questioning about the baby's day and a free ranging discussion of pregnancy and birth. For Daws an important issue is how the mother is able to handle issues connected with separation and attachment. She believes that the issues have to be resolved to allow the mother to begin to distance herself from the child and allow him or her to go to sleep on their own. Daws outlines a number of cases to illustrate the complex and varied nature of the problem, as well as the different methods of treatment. She comments that her treatment involves assisting parents to 'speculate on what the sleeping problems represent in their own child's emotional life and the relationship between them and their child. Understanding this often enables parents to make effective changes' (p. 95). She suggests that there are no automatic solutions but that each problem has to be looked at afresh. Unfortunately, there do not appear to be any studies of the effectiveness of psychoanalytic approaches.

Methodological issues

There appear to have been surprisingly few methodologically sound studies of the effects of treating children with sleeping difficulties. The best conducted studies are those that have involved drug treatment and these have found the weakest effects. The investigations of the behavioural management approach, at first sight, appear to indicate that this method is reasonably effective. However, there are a number of indications that this common assumption should be questioned. Most studies have reported success in only about half the cases. The percentage of successful cases for various studies is as follows: Chavin and Tinson (1980), 56 per cent; Jones and Verduyn (1983), 53 per cent; only 53 per cent entered Richman *et al.*'s (1985) treatment condition; of these 77 per cent showed an improvement; Largo and Hunziker (1984), 85 per cent, Seymour *et al.* (1983) report a success rate of 82 per cent over 6 months; while Weir and Dinnick (1988) found that about half of the children in treatment and control groups improved their sleeping.

It is particularly worrying that the two studies which have employed control groups have not clearly established the effectiveness of behavioural management approaches to treatment. Seymour *et al.* (1989) were able to show that treatment (both advice and booklet) significantly reduced the number of night wakings, but the children after treatment were still waking up, on average, nearly once a night. It is worth noting that in this study the control group showed no improvement and that there was only a four-week gap between pre- and post-treatment measures. In contrast, Weir and Dinnick (1988) found that both treatment and control groups improved from a pre-test to a six-month later post-test. In this study the control group received the normal advice and were referred to other professionals in the usual manner.

These studies raise a number of important issues for consideration. Can we expect sleep problems to spontaneously improve? Because longitudinal studies show a consistent percentage of children above preschool age who have sleeping problems, this at first sight suggests there is a group of children who have persistent sleeping problems and there is little spontaneous improvement. However, a more careful examination of the evidence from longitudinal studies suggests that about half the children can be expected to show a reduction in these problems between any two age points. Before outlining these studies, it should be noted that age differences in the definition of sleeping problems may change the apparent rate of sleeping problems, especially if such definitions are influenced by parental report. If we look at the percentage of children with sleep problems whose later sleeping improves without treatment, then longitudinal studies give the following figures: 59 per cent improve between eight months and three years (Zuckerman *et al.*, 1987); 56 per cent improve between six and twelve months, 59 per cent between twelve and eighteen months, 46 per cent between eighteen months and two years, 71 per cent between two and three years, and 86 per cent improve between three and four and a half years (Jenkins *et al.*, 1984). Thus, one should treat with great caution claims for the effectiveness of treatments which do not use a control group, use older preschool children, and do not take into account the possibility of spontaneous rates of remission. This is of particular concern as many studies have failed to produce high rates of success (see above).

What are the explanations of this pattern of 'spontaneous improvement'? One possibility is that the collection of data will have an effect on the parents' behaviour. Largo and Hunziker suggest that completing sleep diaries will lead to parents becoming aware of the inconsistencies and deficiencies in their behaviour, and this will mean they will adopt more successful strategies. Their own evidence backs up this claim. However, Richman *et al.*, found a weaker effect (11 per cent improved). Thus, although the evidence for the position is not strong, it should be kept in mind. In particular, one might predict that the more detailed the information that parents have to supply and the more prominent sleeping issues are in this account, the more likely is it for parents to adopt new and successful strategies to deal with sleeping problems. It is also the case that if this effect is occurring then a likely consequence is to make it more difficult to identify effective treatment.

Another explanation of spontaneous improvement is that it is not spontaneous in the sense of simply being a result of the maturation of the child's behaviour, but a result of an explicit change in parental strategy. Parents in control groups or longitudinal investigations are not necessarily passive participants in the study of sleeping difficulties. Some are likely to seek out advice from relations, friends, health professionals, and books. Thus, 'spontaneous improvement' may be due to parents adopting successful strategies based on the advice they obtain. It is of particular interest that Seymour *et al.* (1989) found no improvement in a control group over a short period of four weeks, and these families presumably knew they would soon enter a treatment programme – a position which might induce helplessness. In contrast, the control families in the Weir and Dinnick (1988) study received 'normal' advice from their health visitor, nearly half were referred to other health professionals, and the time between assessments was six months; the sleeping pattern of this control group improved. Thus, spontaneous improvements may depend on parental expectations of future help, and the provision of help and support from interested health professionals.

The findings about improvement from longitudinal studies are also interesting in that the rate of this is high but does not change appreciably with an increasing age gap between the points at which data are collected. Such a finding is doubly surprising when one remembers that longitudinal studies find that the actual rate of sleeping difficulties remains at somewhere between a fifth and a third of families during the preschool years (see Messer and Richards, chapter 8). If there is a rate of about 50 per cent 'spontaneous' improvement over time then one would expect a large decrease in the overall rate of sleeping difficulties with increasing age.

How can this contradiction be explained? One obvious explanation is that new sleeping difficulties emerge and so there may be improvement for some families but there is also a deterioration for others. For example, Zuckerman *et al.* (1987) report that of the children at eight months who did not have sleep problems, 26 per cent had sleep problems at three years. Such changes may keep the proportion of children with sleeping difficulties at about the same level. More extensive information is given by Jenkins *et al.* They found that the children who did not have a sleeping problem at 12 months were highly *unlikely* to develop a problem at 18 or 24 months, and that 99/150 children did not have a sleeping problem at any of these three ages. For the remaining children there was a probability between 0.41 to 0.59 (depending on age and classification of whether or not there was a sleeping problem) that their sleeping would improve or become worse. It is notable that only 5 per cent of children had a persistent sleep problem at all three ages. Thus, it would seem that there may be a core of children who do not have sleeping problems, but that for the remainder there is a constant fluctuation of improvement and deterioration. As a result, the percentage of children with sleep problems may remain constant in the early school years, but the individuals who have a problem may change from age point to age point. Such findings point to the need to establish long-term improvement in any treatment study.

What needs to be determined is the reason why some children consistently do not have sleep problems while other children's sleeping is much more inconsistent. This probably involves a consideration of long-term issues (see Messer and Richards, chapter 8), such as child care practice, and infant and parental characteristics. There is also a need to determine what the main factors are that lead to temporary improvement or deterioration of children's sleeping; is it the presence of certain stresses (e.g. new siblings, illnesses, entering nursery) or a result of changes in parental behaviour?

Another issue in the evaluation of sleeping problems is that the large number of advice books on this topic might lead to an overall reduction in the general incidence of these problems, but those that remain may be relatively more difficult to solve. Such considerations make it particularly important to place this research about treatment within the current climate of attitudes to child rearing and the availability of advice to parents about solutions to these problems.

Thus, there still remains a question over the effectiveness of the behavioural management approach to treatment. Further controlled investigations need to be conducted to establish whether this method is successful over the long term. Furthermore, it may be important to consider what features of this or any treatment programme make it effective – is it the availability of certain forms of information (as in information booklets)? Is it the availability of someone who can offer support (as in telephone contacts)? Or it is necessary to have a therapist who can offer strategies tailored to the needs of particular families? In terms of cost-effectiveness of health services it makes sense to consider whether an integrated and progressive service should be offered to families: from information booklets and the use of a self-administered sleep diary to more specific counselling and support, and then to more individual therapy. Furthermore, the possibility of preventative interventions (see Hewitt and Galbraith, 1987) needs to be considered in the future research agenda.

References

Chavin, W. and Tinson, S. (1980), 'Children with sleep difficulties', *Health Visitor*, 53, pp. 477–80.

Daws, D. (1985a), 'Sleep problems in babies and young children', *Journal of Child Psychotherapy*, 11, pp. 87–95.

Daws, D. (1985b), *Through the Night: Helping parents and sleepless infants* (London: Free Association Books).

Douglas, J. and Richman, N. (1982), *Sleep Management Manual* (Institute of Child Health), revised 1985.

Douglas, J. and Richman, N. (1984), *My Child Won't Sleep* (Harmondsworth: Penguin).

Ferber, R. (1986), *Solve Your Child's Sleep Problems* (London: Dorling Kindersley).

Guedeney, A. and Kreisler, L. (1987), 'Sleep disorder in the first 18 months of life: hypothesis on the role of mother–child emotional exchanges', *Infant Mental Health Journal*, 8, pp. 307–18.

Hewitt, K.E. and Galbraith, C.R. (1987), 'Post-natal classes on prevention of sleeplessness in young children', *Child: Care, Health and Development*, 13, pp. 415–20.

Illingworth, R.S. (1987), *The Development of the Infant and Young Child: Normal and Abnormal* (E & S Livingston).

Jenkins, S., Owen, C., Bax, M. and Hart, H. (1984), 'Continuities of common behaviour problems in preschool children', *Journal of Child Psychology and Psychiatry*, 25, pp. 75–89.

Jones, D.P.H. and Verduyn, C.M. (1983), 'Behavioural management of sleep problems', *Archives of Disease in Childhood*, 58, pp. 442–4.

Largo, R.H. and Hunziker, U.A. (1984), 'A developmental approach to the management of children with sleep disturbances in the first three years of life', *European Journal of Paediatrics*, 142, pp. 170–3.

Leach, P. (1989), *Baby and Child* (Harmondsworth: Penguin).

Ousted, M.K. and Hendrick, A.M. (1977), 'The first-born child: patterns of development', *Developmental Medicine and Child Neurology*, 19, pp. 446–53.

Richman, N. (1985), 'A double-blind drug trial of treatment in young children with waking problems', *Journal of Child Psychology and Psychiatry*, 26, pp. 591–8.

Richman, N., Douglas, J., Hunt, H., Lansdown, R. and Levere, R. (1985), 'Behavioural methods in the treatment of sleep disorders – a pilot study', *Journal of Child Psychology and Psychiatry*, 26, pp. 581–90.

Russo, R., Gururaj, V. and Allen, J. (1976), 'The effect of diphenhydramine HCL in paediatric sleep disorders', *Journal of Clinical Pharmacology*, 16, pp. 284–8.

Sanger, S., Weir, K. and Churchill, E. (1981), 'Treatment of sleep problems: the use of behavioural modification techniques by health visitors', *Health Visitor*, 54, pp. 421–2.

Scott, G. and Richards, M. (1989), 'Night waking in infants: effects of providing advice and support for parents', *Journal of Child Psychology and Psychiatry*, 31, pp. 551–67.

Seymour, F.W. (1987), 'Parent management of sleep difficulties in young children', *Behaviour Change*, 4, pp. 39–48.

Seymour, F.W., Bayfield, G., Brock, P. and During, M. (1983), 'Management of night-waking in young children', *Australian Journal of Family Therapy*, 4, pp. 217–23.

Seymour, F.W., Brock, P., During, M. and Poole, G. (1989), Reducing sleep disruptions in young children: evaluation of therapist-guided and written information approaches: a brief report', *Journal of Child Psychology and Psychiatry*, 30, pp. 913–18.

Simonoff, E.A. and Stores, G. (1987), 'Controlled trial of trimeprazine tartrate for night waking', *Archives of Disease in Childhood*, **62**, pp. 253–7.

Spock, B. (1969), *Baby and Child Care* (London: New English Library).

Valman, H.B. (1989), *The First Year of Life* (London: British Medical Association).

Weir, and Dinnick, (1988), 'Behaviour modification in the treatment of sleep problems occurring in young children: a controlled trial using health visitors as therapists', *Child: Care, Health and Development*, **14**, pp. 355–67.

Zuckerman, B., Stevenson, J. and Bailey, V. (1987), 'Sleep problems in early childhood: continuities, predictive factors, and behavioral correlates', *Pediatrics*, **80**, pp. 664–71.

Chapter 11

An overview of infant crying, feeding and sleeping problems

David Messer, Gillian Harris
and Ian St. James-Roberts

One purpose of the original study group was to examine the possibility that crying, feeding and sleeping problems are inter-related; that similar criteria are employed to define a problem; that there are similar or related developmental paths; that there are common causes, and that similar forms of treatment are effective. This chapter follows this division by considering four topics: definition and prevalence, developmental course, causes and treatments. For each topic we bring together the material that has been reviewed in previous chapters. This enables a broader perspective to be provided about the nature of the problems and enables insights to be gained about important developmental characteristics of the problems.

Definition and prevalence

What similarities and differences can be identified in the definitional and formal characteristics of the three problem areas? In many respects, crying and sleeping are the two most similar areas. This conclusion is reached by examining the three areas in terms of: behavioural features; methods of identification; prevalence and seriousness.

Behavioural features

Although infant feeding problems may result in crying or poor sleeping, they may also encompass disturbances in a broad range of other areas of behaviour. For example, infant feeding problems can include failure to thrive (growth problems), food refusal or 'faddiness' and difficulties of ingesting or tolerating food.

In contrast, crying and sleeping problems refer to specific types of behaviour. Even so, they are difficult to define in terms of simple behaviour frequencies or durations. For crying, the amplitude, duration, frequency, pitch and pattern can all vary. For sleeping, the frequency, length, distribution and time of sleep periods, ease of settling and resettling, and behaviour while awake, can all vary.

Atypical crying is the common feature of both sleeping and crying problems. The difference between these two problem areas lies not in the type of infant behaviour, so much as in the age, time of day and context in which the crying occurs. That is, crying problems occur most commonly in 1–3-month-old infants during the evening and afternoon, while sleeping problems occur around settling or waking at night-times in older infants. A distinction can also be drawn between the *amount* and *organisation* of infant sleeping. Although the available evidence is inadequate, it appears that sleeping problems generally have at least as much to do with the organisation of sleeping (that is, with poor settling and waking at night-time) as with sleep deficits.

Methods of identification and measurement

Crying and sleeping problems are usually identified by parents, who may seek professional assistance because of their concerns. As a consequence, issues arise about the subjectivity of parents' reports. There is evidence, for instance, that parents of firstborns are more likely to consider crying a problem and to seek help for it. Likewise, there are well-documented findings that parents vary in what they consider to be a sleeping difficulty, and their standards change with the age of the child. As noted elsewhere in this book, this implies the need to understand how and why parents' views vary, as well as to measure infant behaviour norms.

In view of these differences of opinion among parents, as well as among clinicians and researchers, it is heartening that broadly consistent assessments of problem sleeping and crying behaviour seem to be emerging. That is, there is reasonably good agreement between maternal and tape-recorded measures of crying (Chapter 1), and between maternal and objective assessments of sleeping (infra-red and movement-based (Scher *et al.*, 1992)). It also is reassuring that factor analysis has identified dimensions which contain related sleep problem behaviours (Messer *et al.*, 1992).

As a result, the 'rule of threes' – crying and fussing for at least three hours a day for three or more days a week – can be regarded as a useful rule of thumb for identifying problem crying. Similarly, sleeping problems are often regarded as occurring when a child wakes repeatedly each night for three or more nights a week. As noted above, these 'rule of thumb' definitions should not be adhered to slavishly – other factors, such as crying intensity and the number, quality and duration of wakings, need to be taken into account. However, they provide workable and helpful guidelines for research and practice.

Feeding problems are also usually identified by parental assessments of amount of food ingested, growth faltering, age-inappropriateness of feeding skills (e.g. ability to feed self, intake restricted to liquid or puréed foods), the length of time taken to feed, and the number and severity of behaviour problems occurring at mealtimes (e.g. food refusal, holding food in mouth, vomiting).

Feeding problems differ from crying and sleeping problems in that they may be picked up by routine community screening for growth and weight. Growth faltering is usually best described as a movement down across one or more centile lines. Intake can also be compared with dietary norms for children of comparable height and weight. It is therefore possible to say not only that a child is failing to grow at the expected rate, but also that he or she is not eating the required calories for growth to occur. The widespread use of screening charts for growth and calorie-intake provides a degree of formality in the assessment of feeding problems which is lacking in the other areas.

Prevalence

Using the 'rule of threes' definition of crying, it appears that around a quarter of 1–3-month-old English babies cry for three or more hours in a day, but we do not yet know how many of these consistently cry this much, that is, for three or more days in a week. Presumably, the prevalence is lower. Around 15 to 20 per cent of English mothers seek health service help for the crying, but this rate depends partly on the services available. Beyond three months, the rates halve to 10 per cent or less.

Using the definition of waking several times a night for three or more nights a week (see above) about a fifth of infants have sleeping problems in the latter part of the first year and the second year. Similarly, around a fifth to a third of 2–5 year olds are considered by their parents to have sleeping problems.

The prevalence of feeding problems varies according to type and severity. Most children of toddler age are reported as being 'faddy' to some degree about which foods they will or will not accept. Many parents regard such behaviour as normal and do not seek professional assistance in dealing with it. Forsyth *et al.* (1985) found that one third of mothers in their sample perceived their infants to be difficult to feed in the first three months. However, a study of the prevalence of feeding problems in the general population of Sweden found a rather low rate of acknowledged feeding problems (of 1.4 per cent) in 3–12-month-old infants (Dahl and Sunderlin, 1986). Similarly, there is variation in the reported incidence of non-organic failure to thrive, which ranges from 1 to 5 per cent, according to the definition of growth faltering used and the population being studied.

Location and seriousness of the problem

Although little is currently known about the longer-term outcome of crying and sleeping problems, it appears that the child's behaviour is usually a more important cause of difficulties for the parents than for the child: the child's health and development are not usually seriously at risk. There may, however be indirect consequences for the child, where parent–infant relationships deteriorate sufficiently for neglect or abuse to occur.

Feeding problems may also be mainly a concern for parents, particularly if they are transient. They become serious problems for both parents and infant if they persist and result in growth deficit or if the infant's diet is lacking in specific nutrients. Feeding problems may also act as triggers for abuse of the infant by the parent.

A number of different forms of organic and non-organic failure to thrive are hypothesised to exist. However, their definitions are based on assumptions about the aetiology of the condition, which are controversial. Most infants with failure to thrive gain weight when hospitalised, suggesting that inadequate calorie intake is the immediate cause (see Harris, chapter 6). Measures of calorie intake and growth provide powerful tools for distinguishing serious feeding problems. At present, comparable indices are lacking in the other two areas.

Summary

There are noteworthy differences in the way crying, feeding and sleeping problems are conceptualised and defined. Feeding problems are more readily evaluated and, if sustained, are more serious, because of their impact upon growth. There is currently little evidence that crying or sleeping problems hamper growth or development, so that in the majority of cases these are more obviously problems for parents than for infants. This optimistic prognosis must, however, be qualified by the dearth of longitudinal data on the outcomes in such cases.

Progress has occurred towards criteria and measurements which define problems, albeit rather broadly, within each area. It is estimated that around a fifth of English mothers seek professional assistance for infant crying, while around a quarter of infants cry and fuss for three or more hours in a day at the peak crying age. A third of mothers report their infant as difficult to feed in the first four months and some 1 to 5 per cent can be identified as suffering from non-organic failure to thrive. A number of studies have consistently found that somewhere between a fifth and a third of families report sleeping difficulties in preschool children. A significant minority of infants experience difficulties in all three behaviour areas, but the rate of such composite problems is unknown.

Developmental patterns

As already noted, there are differences in the ages at which crying, feeding and sleeping problems most often occur. It is helpful and instructive to examine the developmental course of the three behaviours in more detail, since such an outline can give clues about aetiology and alert us to links between behaviours. This leads on to an examination of the typical developmental continuity for each problem and of inter-relations between the problems.

The development of crying, feeding and sleeping

What are the major features of the development of crying, feeding and sleeping? Even before birth, the basis of the later sleep cycles can be identified in the foetus (see Zaiwalla and Stein, chapter 7). There is uncertainty whether a foetus can be thought of as having a sleep/wake pattern, mainly because the physiological indices are different from those in a child or adult. At birth, infants spend about two thirds of their time asleep. With increasing age, more time is spent awake. During the first week the longest period asleep is about four hours.

Crying and feeding are established soon after birth, although it usually takes some days before infants adapt to the nipple and to the liquid flow provided by their source of milk. Crying and feeding, like sleeping, are cyclical behaviours which are under neurophysiological control, but are shaped by the demands of the environment.

From birth the amount of crying gradually increases, although it is not yet known whether there is a diurnal pattern of crying in the first few days. It seems likely that soon after birth infants take equal-sized feeds and that there is little diurnal patterning to this behaviour. The mothers' reactions to breast-feeding before six weeks appear important, because this age is the crucial one for the change to bottle feeding. It is, perhaps, no coincidence that crying shows a peak at around six weeks, when infants will often cry for two hours or more per day. What is less clear is the direction of influence between crying, feeding and other processes. At six weeks there is some progress to longer periods of sleep and for more sleep to occur at night.

Thus, our present state of knowledge suggests that in the days immediately after birth infant behaviours show, at most, rudimentary tuning to diurnal rhythms; crying, feeding and sleeping tend to occur irrespective of the time on the clock.

During the first months infants seem to be able to move towards the regulation of calorie intake to accord with growth velocity (see Drewett, chapter 4). This regulation cannot, however, be described as complete. Infants will increase or decrease intake with variation in the caloric density of the feed, but the change in intake will not compensate entirely for the change in caloric density. What is not yet clear is whether or not the mechanisms for regulating hunger and thirst are separate in the neonate. It might seem that the need for water is satisfied by the infant's intake of milk, but there is little evidence to show that neonates respond to a thirst stimulus by increasing their intake of water.

Between two to four months the presence of diurnal cycles in crying, feeding and sleeping becomes increasingly evident. For example, two-month-old bottle-fed infants have their largest intake at the start of the day, whereas breast-fed infants tend to have the largest intake during the afternoon. Crying is concentrated in the afternoon and evening. Most two month olds sleep more in the night than during the day.

After three months crying declines to about an hour per day. The reduction in crying is most marked in the morning, afternoon and evening, with crying still occurring at similar, generally low, rates at night. The 3–4 months age also seems to be a time when infants are maximally sensitive to new tastes (Harris *et al.*, 1990). Solid food tends to be introduced earlier in bottle-fed than breast-fed infants, and often a reason given for the change is the re-occurrence of night waking. By 3–4 months most infants have started to sleep reliably through the night.

Crying problems may continue during the first year, but between 4–12 months only 10 per cent of English mothers seek professional help for this problem. Growth faltering associated with non-organic causes typically seems to begin between three and nine months, depending upon when solid foods are introduced. It is also dependent upon whether or not the milk feed provided before the introduction of solid food is sufficient to maintain growth on the original growth trajectory. Growth faltering is therefore associated with the transition from milk to solid food diet. Problems with the acceptance of new tastes and textures, food refusal and food intolerance are also.associated with this transitional period. Sleeping problems are a greater cause of parental concern during the later half of the first year, and at this age the problems are often brought to the notice of health professionals.

In children who have not had feeding problems in the first year, food faddiness might appear in the second year, and is probably best described as the accession to the age of autonomy, the desire to say 'no', rather than as a feeding problem. The use of transitional objects which are associated with sleeping (blankets, toys put in the bed, etc.) becomes more noticeable in the second year. In children over two or three years, problems with sleeping now include difficulties over bedtime and nightmares, which are rarely reported before this age.

It can be seen that from birth there is a progressive organisation of crying, feeding and sleeping rhythms. The first difficulties are usually associated with infants' adaptation to their mode of feeding. Excessive crying is not usually identified as a problem in the first week or so, and parents usually tolerate the lack of night-time sleeping. Problems with crying become prominent from six weeks, a time when there may be a change from breast- to bottle-feeding, and are common until 12 weeks. By 3–4 months growth faltering without organic cause starts to be noticed and is associated with the introduction of solids. This is the age when professional help is usually sought. By 3–4 months the majority of infants sleep through the night. In the case where this does not occur parents typically become concerned in the second half of the first year. Food refusal becomes a feature of some children's feeding in the second year and sleeping problems can continue from early in the first year until the school years.

Continuities in the development of crying, feeding and sleeping

Infant crying, feeding and sleeping problems show different developmental patterns. Crying in the first three or four months shows moderate levels of stability; infants who cry a lot at one age are likely to cry a lot at another age. Beyond four months there continues to be some predictability into the first year of life, with 'fussing' or irritable behaviour being more stable than crying. Crying problems are unlikely to persist beyond the first year, and infants do appear to 'grow out' of this problem. However, there is some evidence that early persistent crying is associated with other behavioural problems at later ages.

Stable individual differences seem to be present in some dimensions of feeding. Nipple refusals during feeding in the first two days of life predict weight gain during the first month. Sucking characteristics in infants who have been changed from breast- to bottle-feeding predict adiposity during the preschool years (but not after six years). If feeding problems persist through and beyond the first year, then they are unlikely to be resolved without intervention. The problems are likely to continue as difficulties for parents unless growth faltering is present.

Sleeping problems are highly likely to persist up to and beyond the early school years. Several lines of evidence point to sleeping difficulties being unstable; the problem may be reduced or disappear for some time, only to re-emerge at a later age. In his review Stevenson (chapter 9) does not find that sleeping problems are strongly linked with clinical disturbances. Neither do difficulties appear to be associated with widespread behavioural problems at the same age or at later ages (some studies even find a link with higher cognitive abilities at later ages).

Inter-relationships in the development of crying, feeding and sleeping problems

Do crying, feeding and sleeping problems occur together in the same infants? This central question goes beyond the broad issue of resemblances in the behaviour areas to require studies which assess concurrent or successive correlations of the problems within particular infants. As Drewett and Wright have noted (chapters 4 and 5), there is no doubt that parents assume links of this kind. The switch from breast-feeding which occurs at around six weeks of age, for example, is commonly explained in terms of infant crying due to dissatisfaction with breast milk. The question, then, is whether this assumption is correct: do the switched infants cry more than other infants at the same age, and is there evidence that they are really hungry? Similarly, although a link clearly exists between sleeping problems and crying, since this is an element in identifying such problems, it is also possible to ask whether infants who sleep badly are distinguished by high overall crying.

Unfortunately, the overwhelming finding of the present review is that few scientifically controlled studies have examined more than one behaviour area at a time, while those which have done so have concentrated on general community samples rather than cases selected for one or other problem type. To some extent, this may reflect the different concerns of the professional groups involved in this area, as well as the cost of suitable research. Studies of the correlation between crying and sleeping problems, for example, require longitudinal designs which follow the same infants over at least the first two years of life. It is hoped that a greater appreciation of this fragmentation will lead to a more integrated approach in the future.

So far as the existing studies do speak to this question, the impression they give is that the links between the three problem types may be less powerful than is often believed. In relation to feeding, there is consistent evidence that method (breast against bottle), interfeed interval and method changes are related to both crying and sleeping. Even so the relationship is a limited one, and this led Barr *et al.* (1989) to conclude that feeding method is a remarkably weak predictor of crying.

Likewise, although a good feed before bedtime is supposed to lead to a good night's sleep, there is little support for this position. The amount of feed and the time until the next feed show a variety of statistical relations (from positive to negative) across individual infants. In a study of 2-, 4- and 8-week-old bottle-fed infants, Harris *et al.* (1992) found no correlation between the amount of milk taken before sleep and subsequent length of sleep. However, there was a positive correlation between the length of night sleep and the amount of milk consumed on waking. Similarly, rice cereal added to the milk of bottle-fed infants does not effect sleeping through the night. Nor does the presence of a continuous source of nutrition from intravenous infusion appear to disrupt or aid the development of sleeping patterns.

Similarly, fussing (though not crying) has consistently been linked with low concurrent amounts of sleeping (Bernal, 1972; Hurry *et al.*, 1991), but the correlation levels, around 0.4, suggest that the relationship is a modest one (Hurry *et al.*, 1991). Over successive ages, the most reliable relationship is between early fussing/irritability and later problem behaviours, but the picture is patchy, with some researchers finding a link between early fussiness and later sleeping problems (Bernal, 1973), and others finding that fussiness is stable, but does not predict sleeping (St. James-Roberts and Plewis, 1992). There have been suggestions of relations between feeding and sleeping. Difficulties in feeding at three months have been found to be associated with failure to sleep through the night (Moore and Ucko, 1957) and Bernal (1973) reported that more frequent feeding in the first ten days was related to sleeping problems at fourteen months.

Taken as a whole, the implication of these findings is that, although crying, feeding and sleeping problems do occur in the same infants, this probably happens in a minority, rather than in most cases. It is possible that the low levels of concordance reflect the limitations of current research methods and, particularly, the use of general community samples, and this proviso needs to be borne in mind. If it is correct, however, this finding that problems in the three areas most often occur separately has important implications for theory, since over-arching variables, such as temperament, are no longer needed to account for the problems. Instead, the focus needs to shift to the specific developmental and contextual factors involved in each type of problem.

Causes: a multifactorial aetiology

The reviews in this volume are uniform in the conclusion that crying, feeding and sleeping difficulties are the result of a variety of different, and often interacting, variables. St. James-Roberts (chapter 2) writes that no simple explanation for persistent crying is likely to be found. Instead, it may be due to a combination of physiological vulnerabilities, maturational processes and parental responsiveness.

Harris (chapter 6) argues that failure to thrive is best seen as a result of poor calorie intake. This may be the result of the infants' inability to regulate intake, the inability to signal hunger and satiety, the parents' inability to respond to infant signals, the past history of feeding, and inabilities related to the mechanical skills of feeding. Parental mood may be implicated in these processes by influencing the responsiveness to infant signals, either by reduction in responsiveness as in depression, or by over-riding signals of hunger and satiety because of anxiety.

Messer and Richards (chapter 8) present a model of sleeping difficulties which seeks to relate infant characteristics, maternal charcteristics and early experiences. They suggest that all these factors may play a part in the development of sleeping difficulties. They do not claim that all these influences exert a uniform effect across different families, rather, for any particular family different patterns of these influences can result in sleeping difficulties.

For both research and practice, these conclusions have important and far-reaching implications. In particular, they imply that while problems in the three areas may sometimes have simple cause and effect explanations this is likely to be true only in a minority of cases. In the majority, it becomes necessary to think in terms of individual pathways of developmental maladaptation, where different factors accumulate and interact together over time. Equally, it follows that the causal pathways may vary between infants, so that a given type of problem may have a different history from one case to the next.

Although clearly indicated by the available evidence, this 'developmental' view of the origins of infant crying, feeding and sleeping problems is a challenging one, since it implies the need to obtain multiple measurements, both concurrently and over time. As Wolke has shown (chapter 3), it is possible to develop suitable assessment methods and they can be tailored to purpose and size. What is needed most immediately is to isolate the main measurement which can be used for both research and practice.

In the remainder of this section, and prior to turning specifically to the issue of treatment, we summarise the main causal approaches which have been proposed in accounting for infant crying, feeding and sleeping problems. Our aim in doing so is not to favour one or another, so much as to provide a list of the factors which may be involved in any particular case. For practical purposes, the list can be used as a set of topics which need to be reviewed for their relevance when assessing the characteristics of a particular case. For both research and practice, the longer-term goal is to refine this list, develop better means of assessment, and to learn more about the relative importance of the various factors under different circumstances.

Looking across the three types of problem it does not appear that there is good evidence for a common aetiology. Instead, we see different patterns and different hypotheses about causes. Parental behaviour has been implicated in all three conditions, but even here there are different proposals about the way it leads to problems. One possible common theme is that the problems are perpetuated by parents doing 'more of the same' rather than reverting to strategies that normalise the situation (e.g. continuing to take a child into the parental bed).

By reviewing hypotheses about the causes of crying, feeding and sleeping difficulties it is possible to illustrate the complexity of the developmental process and the issues that need to be kept in mind when attempting to treat the problems. So far as possible, the approach adopted is to review the different explanations on a topic by topic basis, but it should be noted that the topics overlap.

The problems are a normal part of development

For both crying and sleeping it can be argued that any difficulties are a part of normal development and that the problems reflect one extreme end of a continuum. This is also true of many feeding problems and even non-organic failure to thrive.

Problems with breast-feeding seem to be commonplace for many mothers (Wright, chapter 5). Furthermore, the expectation that breast-feeding should be an enjoyable and relaxed experience may not prepare mothers for the difficulties and discomforts of breast-feeding. In the same way, food faddiness in toddlers can be perceived as part of the normal developmental process, and part of an appropriate assertion of independence.

Sleeping difficulties also appear to be normal in many families. An issue that is often raised by health professionals is whether sleeping difficulties are the result of the abnormal patterns of child care in Western societies. It is often argued that if infants were to sleep with their mother these difficulties would be removed. In reply, it should be noted that there is a vast range of child care practices across the world, so it is difficult to know which are more 'natural' than others. In addition, child care practices should be seen in relation to the whole culture, and they may be adaptive in relation to the various pressures and influences placed on Western mothers.

It is possible that early difficulties with crying, sleeping and feeding could be a product of problems with the normal re-organisation of behaviour between six and twelve weeks (see St. James-Roberts, chapter 2). According to such an account, children who have these problems might cry more or have problems adapting to solid food and night-time sleeping. The evidence to support such a hypothesis is correlational and not yet very strong.

Physiological disturbances

In considering the problems of crying, feeding and sleeping it is rare for a physiological mechanism to be postulated by itself without reference to some environmental influence, such as crying or sleeping problems being caused by the content of milk. Furthermore, when a physiological cause is discussed it is often considered in global terms with little detail being presented about the precise nature of the underlying process.

One relatively 'pure' hypothesis about a physiological mechanism is the idea that crying might be due to gastrointestinal disturbance. However, support for the idea is limited (see St. James-Roberts, chapter 2). Where associations are found, with breath hydrogen levels and motilin levels, it is not clear whether this is a result or a cause of crying. Somewhat clearer is the finding that crying is associated with painful experiences of a minority of infants, and that the pain is linked in some cases to the occurrence of feeds.

Another hypothesis about a physiological cause has been the association between excessive crying and an allergy to cow's milk. There is support for this occurring in a sub-group of infants. However, Wolke (chapter 3) suggests that such infants should be re-challenged at later ages, so that an 'allergic' baby syndrome does not develop. There also are findings which suggest that intolerance to cow's milk is associated with sleeping difficulties in a small proportion of infants.

The development of feeding may involve an optimal period at three to four months for the introduction of food, an age when infants are accepting of different tastes (Harris *et al.*, 1990). If this period is passed then there is likely to be greater difficulty for the child in acquiring a normal eating pattern. Thus, physiological mechanisms may interact with caregiver beliefs and practices in the development of food preferences.

Sometimes failure to thrive can be attributed to mechanical difficulties. Difficulties with swallowing can mean that mealtimes are lengthy, and parents may interpret the slowness as satiation or may terminate feeds earlier than needed. Again, we see that a physiological cause may interact with another factor to produce a particular developmental problem. Alternatively, a child who is metabolically efficient, in needing only a low calorie intake to maintain optimal growth, may be subject to long and coercive mealtime interactions in an attempt by the parents to get the child to eat more than the child wants or needs. Thus, a functioning physiological mechanism which regulates intake to accord with metabolic rate and growth velocity is misperceived by some parents.

There have been reports of a relationship between birth complications and later sleep problems. However, it is not entirely clear whether this is a result of some common physiological mechanism, some physiological consequence of the birth complications, or of alterations of maternal behaviour due to the difficulties and anxieties caused by the birth complications. Given the findings about sleeping, it is surprising that excessive crying has not reliably been found to be associated with birth complications, and more precise studies of this possible link are needed.

Although physiological mechanisms are likely to be an important feature of crying, feeding and sleeping problems there is only limited evidence about the links. The best documented relation concerns the possibility of crying and sleeping problems being related to an allergy to cow's milk, and mechanical difficulties in eating leading to poor weight gain.

Temperament and individual differences

Associations have been detected between difficult temperament and early crying. There are also reports of similar associations for sleeping. Thus, mothers tend to rate infants with such problems as more difficult, but this is unsurprising given the impact that both these behaviours can have on maternal attitudes and perceptions. Perhaps the safest conclusion is that infants who cry a lot and wake at night are perceived to be difficult infants.

A more specific hypothesis is that some infants may have difficulty in dealing with arousing stimuli, i.e. that they are less able to soothe themselves and so regain equilibrium. Findings reveal that some infants are indeed less able than most to deal with stressful situations. What remains to be established is whether these infants are excessive criers and whether such infants have difficulty in settling themselves to sleep.

Individual differences are, as will be discussed later, implicated in the aetiology of non-organic failure to thrive. It has been noted that infants with non-organic failure to thrive are often perceived as making few demands for food. Moreover, it is only some infants from similar circumstances, and even from the same family, who develop the condition. This suggests an interaction between infant characteristics and environmental conditions.

Although, difficult temperament and related characteristics are often thought of as being associated with crying, feeding or sleeping problems, the evidence for such associations is weak. A major methodological problem is identifying infant temperament independently of any difficulties of crying, feeding or sleeping.

Demographic influences

If we move away from processes which can be thought of as internal to the child, we can start to consider the way that the environment may contribute to the aetiology of the problems. The general influences that typically have been considered concern variables such as SES (Socio Economic Status), gender and parity. Gender can also be considered a biological variable, but will be discussed here because of its social and demographic role.

Mothers of firstborn infants are more likely to report difficulties with crying, but there does not seem to be strong or consistent evidence for birth order or gender differences in actual crying. There is an absence of studies examining the relation of SES to crying with any degree of precision.

The prevalence of breast-feeding is related to SES, and breast-feeding is associated with a slightly higher prevalence of sleeping problems (interestingly, there is not a strong association between SES and sleeping). In specific ethnic groups in the United Kingdom, there is a cultural norm for bottle-feeding and the late introduction of solids. This is associated with the faltering of growth and the comparatively late acquisition of feeding skills.

The relation between demographic information and sleeping difficulties has been analysed in a number of studies. Sleeping difficulties, unlike most childhood difficulties, are not strongly related to SES (see Messer and Richards, chapter 8; Pollock, 1992), to the gender of the infant, or to parity.

Demographic factors have a major influence on many child characteristics and many problems of development are associated with SES and gender. Although demographic variables are sometimes found to be associated with crying and sleeping difficulties they are usually weak predictors.

Learning and parent–child interaction

There are a number of different ways in which experiences can influence the development of problematic behaviour. The most simple mechanism is that learning experience, not dependent on adult behaviour, can result in behavioural difficulties. For example, food refusal or faddiness can sometimes be attributed to the association of food with nausea and vomiting, or with aversive mealtime interactions between parent and child. More prevalent is the suggestion that parental responses play a part in initiating or at least maintaining the difficulties. There is also the suggestion that the actual relationship between mother and child may emotionally affect the child and lead to failure to thrive.

The view that crying is the result of *inadequate* parental responsiveness derives from Bowlby's attachment theory, and was proposed by Bell and Ainsworth (1972). The theoretical basis of this proposal was criticised by Gewirtz and Boyd (1977). More recent work by Hubbard and van IJzendoorn (1991) has indicated that a delay in maternal response is weakly associated with a *decreased* frequency of later crying, and no significant relationship was found with the duration of crying. Furthermore, as St. James-Roberts (chapter 2) argues, it is not clear why parental responsiveness should produce an evening crying peak and a peak in crying at six weeks.

Because feeding difficulties cover a wide range of behaviour, several accounts have been put forward to explain their development. The difficulties with breast-feeding have been attributed not just to the problems of adapting to the characteristics of the mother's nipple and milk supply, but also to the possibility that breast-feeding become *aversive* due to infants being forced onto the breast.

Other forms of feeding difficulty, particularly with solid food, have been explained as due to parents ignoring infants' signals of satiety and thereby making feeding a coercive and unpleasant process. Growth faltering is sometimes thought to be caused by parents ignoring an infant's 'weak' signals of hunger. In addition, there is the possibility that the stress and tension associated with feeding in some families will make it an aversive process. Here the causal mechanism is usually seen as the *negative* events associated with feeding.

Social learning may also play a part in the development of feeding patterns. There is evidence that seeing others eat a new food encourages children to try it. Children who are difficult to feed are frequently fed by themselves and not at family mealtimes, and they therefore have no opportunity to observe and imitate normal eating behaviour. There is also an argument that food preferences can be altered by the way that food is implicitly valued by adults (eat up A so that you can have B, implies B is more pleasurable than A); here social and cognitive processes are implicated.

A common viewpoint is that sleeping difficulties are caused by parental *responsiveness*. According to this account, parents reinforce children's wakings by their responses and attention. As a result, the behaviour is maintained. It may also be that parents become the *discriminative stimulus* for sleeping to occur, and as a result need to be present for a child to fall asleep. In addition, learning theory has been used to stress the need for routines to occur so that these provide the cues for sleep.

In the feeding literature the possibility that a poor *mother–infant relation-ship* can cause failure to thrive has been a prominent orientation. It is supposed that infants' depressive emotional response to a poor relationship may lead to loss of appetite or hormonal deficiency (Oates, 1984). A distinction is sometimes made between early onset non-organic failure to thrive, which has been suggested to be the result of insecure attachment formation between mother and infant, and a later onset food refusal caused by the mother's inability to allow the child autonomy and the regulation of his or her own intake.

Maternal depression affects mother–infant social interaction (Murray and Stein, 1989) and is associated with crying, feeding and sleeping problems. Depression is not only associated with excessive crying, but when the crying is reduced so is the depression (Pritchard, 1986). Reports of physical difficulties with breast-feeding have been found to be higher in mothers who are depressed, and these mothers stop breast-feeding earlier. Maternal depression also has been found to be associated with sleeping difficulties. However, the causal mechanism is not clear, in that maternal depression may lead to infant behavioural difficulties or infant behavioural difficulties may lead to depression.

The possibility that parental behaviour is a cause of crying, feeding and sleeping problems has received considerable attention, and at first sight this appears to give coherence across the three areas. However, a closer consideration of the causal mechanisms reveals that very different types of parental behaviour are implicated in the aetiology of the three conditions. For crying, the lack of responsiveness has been claimed as a cause, for feeding the negative nature of parental behaviour or the experience of food has been emphasised, and for sleeping (and sometimes crying) the rewarding of the behaviour by parental response has been emphasised.

Treatment

The treatment of the three types of problem can broadly be classified in terms of either direct interventions, such as the use of drugs and hospitalisation, or modifications of child and, more usually, parental behaviour. Before going on to discuss these two areas it is worth noting that there have been studies of methods which will immediately lead to a reduction in crying or send a baby to sleep, such as rocking, use of pacifier and rhythmical noises. As Wolke (chapter 3) observes, however, there is little evidence that such interventions provide an effective cure for babies who are already high criers.

Direct interventions

The use of antispasmodic drugs to treat infant colic has been found to reduce the amount of crying during and after administration (see chapter 3).

However, the rate of crying after treatment is still higher than normal, and it has been questioned whether the effect of the drug occurs because of the reduction in colic or because of some effect on the CNS. Furthermore, in these studies a notable number of infants improved in the placebo condition.

Perhaps the most direct intervention for growth faltering is the use of naso-gastric feeds. These are undoubtedly effective in helping children to increase their weight. However, Harris (chapter 6) has criticised the method for being counter-productive in the establishment of normal feeding patterns, and in making the problem of food refusal worse. Similar long-term difficulties may occur with high calorie supplements.

Sleeping difficulties are reduced while drugs are administered to the child; children fall asleep more quickly and sleep for longer periods. However, several carefully controlled studies have found that sleeping difficulties re-occur when the drug is no longer administered.

Thus, across all three areas direct interventions do not seem to stop the behavioural problem. An implication of this is that the problem is a product of either the child's characteristics or of the child's interactions with the environment; attempts to simply stop the behaviour may not lead to a solution because alternative, more effective patterns of behaviour are not acquired.

Alteration of infant and maternal activities

Interventions involving parental behaviour are the primary treatment method in all three areas. This is often taken as evidence that parental behaviour is the cause of the problem, but this is not necessarily the case. The concept of special environmental needs (chapter 2) argues that some infants have needs for environmental support and regulation beyond those of most infants. In such cases, parental care which goes further than that which most parents and infants find satisfactory may provide an effective treatment.

For all three types of problem, the most common way to attempt to change infant and maternal activities involves the behavioural management approach. However, there are examples of other methods, which have been tried because of theoretical beliefs or because of the technique has been observed to be used successfully by some mothers.

For example, it has been found that extra physical contact reduces the amount of crying in young infants. Unfortunately, this has not proved reliable or to be an effective intervention for infants who have already been identified as crying excessively by their parents. Studies which have attempted to reduce parental stimulation in an effort to reduce crying have met with mixed success. Sometimes the use of differential reinforcement appears to reduce the amount of crying, but there is no evaluation of this method with a sample which has a satisfactory size.

A successful behavioural management approach to crying in the early months has been carried out by Wolke and his colleagues (see Wolke, chapter

3). The intervention provided information as well as involving therapists in problem solving. This was more successful than an empathy counselling process or a control group when crying was evaluated three months later.

The effectiveness of behavioural management programmes with feeding problems has usually been evaluated without the use of control groups. The findings from these studies suggest that improvements usually occur, but the methodological shortcomings mean caution should be exercised before accepting this conclusion. The basic technique is to reinforce desired behaviours by adult attention, praise, music, stickers, etc. Sometimes the extinction of inappropriate behaviours is attempted by time-out periods which can involve averting eye contact or taking the child to another location. The use of aversive methods has occasionally been employed, the child being ignored until appropriate feeding occurs or, in more extreme circumstances, force feeding is employed. Harris (chapter 6) comments that aversive conditioning is unlikely to continue to be successful once the schedule is terminated.

Another technique used in cases of non-organic failure to thrive is to try to improve maternal sensitivity to infant signals of satiety and hunger. Unfortunately, there have been few investigations of such programmes, and the available evidence suggests that infant's responses to food rather than maternal behaviour have improved.

One other strategy in the treatment of non-organic failure to thrive has been to change the mother's mental state and thereby affect her relationship with her infant. It is assumed that this will affect the feeding process. A study adopting this approach by Iwaniec and Herbert (1988) achieved a high rate of success, but no adequate controls were used in the design. It is possible that attempts to alter mother–infant relationships may result in a better style of feeding, rather than just a change in the emotional climate. Formal evaluations of this possibility need to be made when the effectiveness of such programmes is assessed.

A number of studies have evaluated the success of behavioural management techniques with sleeping difficulties. Generally the studies report somewhere between a half and three-quarters of children improve. Like studies of crying and feeding, most of these investigations suffer from the lack of a control group, so the findings need to be interpreted with caution. This is especially important, as without intervention nearly 50 per cent of parents report improvements in sleeping across age points. A study by Seymour should be noted in that improvements were achieved by the use of information leaflets and this was as effective as counselling (see chapter 10).

Summary

There is still considerable uncertainty about the effectiveness of methods of treatment. The methodologically most satisfactory studies have been concerned with the effects of drugs on crying and sleeping. However, these studies have not provided convincing evidence for the long-term benefits of drug interventions. The direct intervention used with feeding problems also may be ineffective over the long term. Treatments using behavioural management approaches are often, but by no means uniformly, effective and the research literature on crying, feeding and sleeping is plagued by the lack of appropriate control groups. One implication is that when behavioural management approaches are effective this is not simply due to the formal properties of the programme, but due to the sensitivity and problem-solving skills of the therapist.

Overview

A common-sense notion is that the crying of a young infant leads to feeding, the feeding is followed by drowsiness and sleeping; then the cycle can begin again. Such a view suggests that difficulties that occur for one behaviour should also occur for the other behaviours. However, at present we do not have convincing evidence for such links. This may partly be due to the limited research base; there are few studies that have examined the inter-relations between these three behaviours. In the near future we are likely to have fuller answers to these questions as several investigations are analysing or collecting such information. These investigations have, in part, been stimulated by the work for this book!

It has been repeatedly stated that crying, feeding and sleeping problems occur in a significant proportion of children. They are of great concern to parents and, as a result, become an important problem for health professionals. Unfortunately, the research literature does not identify methods of treatment that can be confidently predicted to succeed. In contrast, therapists often have great faith in the particular method of treatment they use. The body of research that we review suggests that their confidence could be misplaced unless there is both an evaluation of the behaviour of the child after treatment, and the rate of success exceeds that in a control group.

An important issue that is scarcely touched on in this review is the possibility of prevention. The findings from cross-cultural studies suggest that parental behaviour may influence the overall amount of crying. If this is correct then it should be possible to identify the parenting styles which can reduce crying. It seems likely that mothers will breast-feed for longer if they are prepared for the problems that occur, and feeding problems could be reduced by making mothers more aware of infants' signals about satiety and hunger. Similarly, it would be sensible to provide expectant mothers with better information about the strategies and routines to adopt when they are dealing with the sleeping of their young baby. Given the uncertainties, cost and unpredictability of treatment much more interest needs to be paid to methods of prevention.

References

Barr, R.G., Kramer, M.S., Pless, I.B., Boisjoly, C. and Leduc, D. (1989), 'Feeding and temperament as determinants of early infant crying/fussing behavior', *Pediatrics*, **84**, pp. 514–21.

Bell, S.M. and Ainsworth, M.D.S. (1972), 'Infant crying and maternal responsiveness', *Child Development*, **43**, pp. 1171–90.

Bernal, J.F. (1972), 'Crying during the first 10 days of life and maternal responses', *Developmental Medicine and Child Neurology*, **14**, pp. 362–72.

Bernal, J.F. (1973), 'Night waking in infants during the first 14 months', *Developmental Medicine and Child Neurology*, **15**, pp. 760–9.

Dahl, M. and Sunderlin, D.C. (1986), 'Early feeding problems in an affluent society', *Acta Paediatrica Scandinavica*, **75**, pp. 380–7.

Forsyth, B.W.C., Leventhal, J.M. and McCarthy, P.L. (1985), 'Mothers' perceptions of problems of feeding and crying behaviors. A prospective study', *American Journal of Disease in Childhood*, **139**, pp. 269–72.

Gewirtz, J.L. and Boyd, E.F. (1977), 'Does maternal responding imply reduced infant crying?', *Child Development*, **48**, pp. 1200–7.

Harris, G., Thomas, A.M. and Booth, D.A. (1990), 'Development of salt taste in infancy', *Developmental Psychology*, **268**, pp. 535–8.

Harris, G., Thomas, A. and Elsdon, H. (1992), 'Feeding, sleeping and crying behaviour in bottle fed infants', in preparation.

Hubbard, F.O.A. and van IJzendoorn, M.H. (1991), 'Maternal unresponsiveness and infant crying across the first 9 months: a naturalistic longitudinal study', *Infant Behavior and Development*, **14**, pp. 299–312.

Hurry, J., Bowyer, J. and St. James-Roberts, I. (1991), 'The development of infant crying and its relationship to sleep–waking organisation', *Society for Research in Child Development Abstracts*, **8**, p. 303.

Iwaniec, D., Herbert, M. and Sluckin, A. (1988), 'Helping emotionally abused children who fail to thrive', in K. Browne, C. Davies and P. Stratton (eds), *Early Prediction and Prevention of Child Abuse* (Chichester: John Wiley).

Messer, D., Richards, M. and Scott, C. (1992), 'Predictors of children's sleeping patterns at 3–4 years of age', Presented at the Annual Conference of the Society of Reproductive and Infant Psychology, Durham, September.

Moore, T. and Ucko, L.E. (1957), 'Night waking in infancy. Part I', *Archives of Disease in Childhood*, **32**, pp. 333–42.

Murray, L. and Stein, A. (1989), 'The effects of postnatal depression on the infant', *Bailliere's Clinical Obstetrics and Gynaeocology*, pp. 921–33.

Oates, R.K. (1984), 'Similarities and differences between nonorganic failure to thrive and deprivation dwarfism', *Child Abuse and Neglect*, **8**, pp. 439–45.

Pollock, J.I. (1992), 'Predictors and long term associations of reported sleeping difficulties in infancy', *Journal of Reproductive and Infant Psychology*, **10**, pp. 151–68.

Pritchard, P. (1986), 'An infant crying clinic', *Health Visitor*, **59**, pp. 375–7.

St. James-Roberts, I. and Plewis, I. (1992), 'Infant behaviour problems: stabilities and links between problems in the first year', Presented at the Annual Conference of the British Psychological Society: Developmental Section, Edinburgh, 11–14 September.

Scher, A., Epstein, R., Sadeh, A., Tirosh, E. and Laurie, P. (1992), 'Toddlers' sleep and temperament: reporting bias or a valid link?', *Journal of Child Psychology and Psychiatry*, **33**, pp. 1249–54.

Index